WOMEN AT RISK

The Real Truth About Sexually Transmitted Disease

[handwritten inscription] Sharon,
through God bless you
really
Phillie   W David Hager

WOMEN AT RISK

*The Real Truth
About Sexually
Transmitted Disease*

DAVID HAGER, M.D.
DONALD JOY, PH.D.

WOMEN AT RISK:
The Real Truth About Sexually Transmitted Disease
Copyright © 1993 by David Hager, M.D. and Donald Joy, PH.D.

First Edition, February 1993

Unless otherwise indicated, all Scripture quotations are from the *Holy Bible, New International Version* © 1973, 1978, 1984 by the International Bible Society. Used by permission of Zondervan Publishing House.

Scripture quotations indicated (NASB) are from the *New American Standard Bible* © 1960, 1962, 1963, 1968, 1971, 1972, 1973, 1975, 1977 by the Lockman Foundation. Used by permission.

ISBN 0-917851-62-5

Printed in the United States of America.

BRISTOL BOOKS
An imprint of Bristol House, Ltd.
2201 Regency Road, Suite 301 • Lexington, KY 40503
Phone: (606) 276-4583
Fax: (606) 276-5365

To order, call our toll-free line: 1-800-451-READ

Contents

Introduction: This Book's for You 7

Chapter One: A Shattered Dream
Case Study: When a Secret Turns into HPV 15

Chapter Two: A Double-Edged Sword
Case Study: When Infidelity Leaves Herpes Tracks 31

Chapter Three: An Emergency in the Sky
Case Study: Self-Pity, Street Sex and Telltale Gonorrhea 45

Chapter Four: One Hot Summer Night
*Case Study: Swinging Sex, Estrangement, Rape
and Chlamydia* 59

Chapter Five: Beside the Old Gray Barn
Case Study: Viral Ripple Effects 73

Chapter Six: Recognizing the Dark Side
Case Study: AIDS and Fatal Attachment 83

Chapter Seven: Silence in the Pool
Case Study: Group B Streptococci, the Stealthy Infection 97

Chapter Eight: A Stolen Briefcase
Case Study: Dealing with Trichomoniasis 107

Chapter Nine: Walking through the Fire
Case Study: Post Abortion Syndrome and Recovery 119

Chapter Ten: Baseball vs. Europe
Case Study: The Loss of Ovaries 131

Chapter Eleven: Confession in a Hotel Room
Case Study: Bacterial Vaginosis 143

Epilogue: A Salute to Heroic Women! 155

Introduction

This Book's for You . . .

"Sexual intercourse is the ultimate expression of my love. It is the most beautiful way for me to express intimacy with the one that I am committed to."

"To say that Christian morality means that I cannot share an expression of my feelings for one that I love through sexual intercourse except in the confines of marriage is prudish and out of touch with reality."

"As a Christian, I am very selective about the person with whom I will be sexually intimate. I don't just sleep around with anyone. People who are promiscuous get venereal diseases; if you are selective and careful you can avoid these types of infections."

These are statements that I have heard in my office in the practice of obstetrics and gynecology. In my life and work as a physician, I speak freely about my personal relationship with Jesus Christ. Consequently, many women who also want to follow Christ seek my services for their medical care. Even some of these women have made statements such as the ones above.

"Shocking!" you say. "Unbelievable!" No. The statements merely reflect the moral and spiritual climate of the days in which we live. God has not called me to pronounce judgment on people who make personal sexual choices based on such rationale. However, I find God often uses me as I communicate with patients and clients from a sound medical perspective which is grounded in my faith. I do not hesitate to explain the grave and irrevocable consequences of a life-style that includes multiple sexual partners.

Some patients with whom I counsel have compartmentalized their sexuality, isolating it from their Christian understanding. They are either unwilling or unable to allow their personal relationship with Christ to have an impact on this area of their lives. Such believers tend to be selective in their obedience to scriptural authority, living by only those Bible teachings that "feel right" or "make sense."

In other cases, a misunderstanding of the whole nature of love is at fault. Love is interpreted as license for full sexual expression regardless of marital status. There seems to be little or no understanding of that aspect of love which is based on moral purity and contains boundaries.

In our society, seeing and wanting something is equated with having what we want. We are all sensitive to basic human "needs," but our self-centeredness tends to confuse "wants" with "needs" and turns them into "my rights." This is one of the reasons why it has been so difficult for us to convince Christian young people that "Saying NO" is the only way to say "YES" to the God-inspired dream of exclusive, life-long sexual intimacy. Abstinence — waiting for sexual intercourse only in marriage — is urgent for saying that big "YES!" In our culture, we give our young people a lot of mixed signals. We do not set a good example for our youth.

Saying 'NO!' to Say 'YES'

If experience is the best teacher, then I am eager to narrate some actual case histories, completely disguised to protect the actual people they represent. Perhaps the information from other's cases maybe applicable in your life. In the Bible God says, "my people are destroyed from lack of knowledge" (Hosea 4:6). My hope is that you will be able to read this medical, developmental and biblical material. We have written it in plain English. This book looks at the Creation which is visible in the female reproductive system, the traumas involved in dealing with unusual pregnancy, reproductive disorders and circumstances that often lead to infection with a sexually transmitted disease (STD). Several chapters deal with STDs, the symptoms and signs that may indicate the presence of an STD, what can be done to treat or control these diseases and what steps are necessary emotionally and spiritually to make the journey toward healing and wholeness.

In my practice of obstetrics and gynecology, patients frequently tell me similar stories about the onset of sexual activity in their lives. Most sexual contact begins in their adolescent years with intermittent episodes of intercourse. Ignorant of the "law of diminishing returns" that pre-

dicts an increased appetite for sexual pleasure, they un-
wittingly whet their appetite for more and more frequent
intercourse with what tends to be an increasing number
of partners.

Walking down the center aisle of a church building in
a white dress and placing a gold band on the finger does
not, to their astonishment, do anything to diminish the
desire for sex with multiple partners. The forbidden fruit
has been tasted and the appetite calls for more. Inevitably sex within marriage becomes routine and predictable; then an emotional quick fix is obtained via a partner
outside the marriage. In the 1990s, such a decision will,
in time, almost certainly bring the female partner to my
office complaining of symptoms consistent with the diagnosis of one of many common STDs prevalent in our
population.

Any gynecologist will confirm that the health risks
posed by the presence of STDs are far greater for the
female population than for the male. Chlamydia and gonorrhea, two of the most frequently seen STDs, can result
in chronic pain, pelvic inflammatory disease, infertility
and permanent damage to the uterus, tubes and ovaries.
Contracting human papilloma virus (HPV) puts women
at far greater risk for certain cancers than men. While
men can develop cancer of the penis as a consequence
of HPV, it is far more common to see cancer of the
cervix and vulva in women who have contracted this
STD.

Often I ask this question, "Do you realize that when
you have intercourse with one partner, you are in es-
sence having sex with everyone with whom that person

has had sex?" If your partner has had even one contact with an infected person, your partner is at risk and may have exposed you to that sexual infection. You become at risk, instantly, to the viruses of all his previous partners.

A patient's usual response to my question is: "No, I was too caught up in the emotion of the moment to think about that." This book is an effort to inform both men and women of the radical, life-altering consequences of a decision that needs to be made in the cool of the day and not in the heat of night-time passion.

More than 10 years ago I agreed to teach a session on sexually transmitted diseases during a "lock-in" for senior high school men at the church where my family and I are members. The youth pastor also had asked Dr. Donald Joy to precede my teaching by describing the world of healthy relationships and lifelong exclusive pair bonding. Each of us listened to the other's session. That was only a beginning of what has turned out to be informal collaboration between Don and me. He frequently refers his counselees to me — both from the area and from Asbury Seminary where he teaches. He has an uncanny ability to sense when there may be a physiological basis for emotional and spiritual problems, so I get some of those referrals.

Across the years, I have come to depend personally on Professor Joy. I am easily captivated by anyone whose presence and words can lift the fog which has seemed to surround some urgent life issue. Indeed, Don's *Unfinished Business: How a Man Can Make Peace with His Past* opened the door for me to bring integrity to my own life in a break-through that is significantly enriching. I'm glad to report that his book on men's issues is now being released in a "recovery shelf" paperback edition, revised, under the title, *Men Under Construction!*

Dr. Joy has a unique ability to capsulize the events surrounding an issue, to put things into perspective and help me to see the answer in a way that makes me feel that I found the solution myself. He has been counselor, encourager and friend to me. It was only natural for me to ask him to provide reflective commentary on the cases which I have compiled from my experience as an obstetrician/gynecologist.

Dr. Joy's research field is human growth and development, especially the fields of epistemology, moral reasoning and faith development. His early research on conscience — objective vs. subjective responsibility — led him to an amazing breakthrough on just how the sexes differ. He has given us a dozen books ranging from moral development insight to sexual development and marriage issues.

Don Joy and I both work from a deep and growing understanding of both "theology" (how God is working in the world) and "psychology" (how the human spirit works). This will not seem like a traditional "religious" book, but it rings true to the deep Christian commitments that shape us. The book will invite you to find a fixed point of reference around which to build your life, too. Since we work on the thesis that our bodies, our sexual behavior and our personalities are wrapped into a solid whole person package, the cases and the reflection on them combine to present a very "spiritual" book in the grandest possible sense.

Dr. Joy was excited about my vision for this book and accepted my invitation to contribute the "reflections" that follow each case. We have both learned a great deal as we have prepared these cases which indicate so dramatically how we are all at risk.

As you read these case scenarios, you may reflect on an event from your past or even your present experience. You may be reminded of a friend who has confronted or is confronting one of these situations. You may have a child who can be helped to avoid making a mistake that could result in lifelong consequences. Whatever your reason for reading these pages, I hope you will be generous in passing along your copy of the book. Give away anything that has been helpful to you.

W. David Hager, M. D., FACOG
Lexington, Kentucky

Chapter One

A Shattered Dream

by W. David Hager, M.D.

I grew up in a small central Kentucky town where athletics played a major role my life during my high school days. I loved sports and played football, basketball and baseball competitively. I certainly was not a great football player, but I did receive inquiries from three colleges about a possible scholarship.

I remember the feeling on those crisp, invigorating fall evenings when the entire community seemed to be in a football frenzy. The attention of my hometown people was directed toward a small group of young men dressed in red and white who played hard and despised losing.

My ambition was to play college football, but it was rudely interrupted one Friday night when I tackled an opposing halfback head on. I hit him too low and his knee caught the back of my neck. For three days I knew nothing. Those around me were uncertain if I would ever be normal again. The severe concussion left me dazed and confused. Over the next four weeks, I recovered. Today I show little evidence of the injury except for the fact that my vision was altered.

Because of the injury, however, I was told to forget about any possibility of playing college football. I was crushed. My dreams shattered, I decided to attend a school that did not even engage in intercollegiate football. In that environment I could completely avoid reminders of my disappointment. I chose a small, Christian college in Wilmore, Kentucky — Asbury College.

I was angry with God for allowing something like this to happen to me. How could he love me and let me be so disappointed? But how could I have known that God would give me unusual opportunities even in my life-shattering disappointment?

If I had not been injured and had not attended Asbury College, God would not have been able to begin a powerful work in my life that is only now beginning to come to full momentum. And if I had not gone to Asbury College I would not have met the most beautiful and talented woman in God's universe. God has used Linda Carruth Hager to enable me to become the man he intended for me to be. She has given birth to and mothered three sons, Philip, Neal and Jonathan, who are the apples of my eye.

I had no idea how an event in my life at 17 years of age would have such a profound effect on all the years to follow. I remembered these events when I heard the story of Sally and Stuart in my office one afternoon.

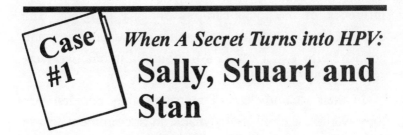

When A Secret Turns into HPV:
Sally, Stuart and Stan

Sally and her sister grew up with their mother in a large, mid-western city after their father left home with another woman. Their mother worked hard to provide the necessities of life for her daughters by holding down two jobs. Needless to say, she was not at home much for interaction with the girls.

Sally Loves Stuart

At 17 years of age, Sally met Stuart, a handsome, energetic young man, and fell in love. They became sexually active as Sally reached out for someone with whom she could be intimate and who would be there for her.

After a one-year relationship, the couple broke up. Shortly thereafter Sally developed numerous wart-like lesions on the outside of the vagina. She went to a family physician who treated her with a solution called trichloracetic acid to chemically eradicate the "genital warts."

Sally Marries Stan

When Sally was 21 years old, she met Stan, a fellow student in night school who reminded her a great deal of Stuart. Sally and Stan dated for a year and decided to get married. Sally had become a Christian as a result of the influence of the local campus ministry program. She brought her fiance with her to many of the activities, and soon he also experienced a profound Christian conversion and abandoned his substance abuse.

In their second year of marriage, they decided that they wanted a child. Sally made an appointment to see me for her pre-pregnancy exam. Her examination was normal by appearance. However, later that week a PAP smear of cells from her cervix returned showing cancer cells. The reading indicated that she had been exposed to human papilloma virus (HPV). The virus that causes genital warts is frequently associated with cervical cancer.

HPV has rapidly become one of the most prevalent STDs in the United States. Although physicians are not required to report all detected cases of this disease, estimates of its prevalence have been made. Recent data indicate that 2.5 to 3 million new cases of HPV occur annually. It is difficult to estimate numbers of cases because many men and women have no symptoms and are totally unaware that they are infected.

The HPV virus can cause visible cauliflower-type warts in the vagina, on the lips of the vagina, the perineum and around the anus in women. Warts usually occur on the shaft of the penis in men but can occur in the urethra as well. A common site of occurrence in gay men is the anus and perianal region. Warts may also be very small, flat lesions which are only visible by searching for them with a microscope. This type of wart is frequently found on the cervix and is associated with the development of pre-cancerous and cancer cells in women.

HPV is transmitted by direct contact with a person who is infected, usually by genital-genital or genital-anal contact. Unlike many STDs, however, HPV has a variable incubation period — the time from exposure until the disease becomes evident. A person who is infected with the virus may develop warts in a few weeks, but it may be months or even years before the lesions become visible. Once infected, the person may never be free of the virus, and recurrences of lesions are not uncommon.

Infected individuals may have some itching and discomfort at the site of the warts, but often the first evidence of infection is the occurrence of the warts themselves. HPV may be diagnosed from a PAP smear or from the biopsy of a wart, but visible lesions are usually diagnosed merely on their appearance. The diagnosis in men can often be made only by using a dilute solution of acetic acid (vinegar) to cause the warts to become white. They can then be visually examined with a microscope or magnifying lens. In women, this solution is placed on the cervix and vulva and in the vagina before performing a microscopic procedure called colposcopy. During colposcopy, the tiny white, raised warts can be seen. Biopsies can then be taken of these areas and sent to a pathologist to confirm the visual diagnosis.

HPV has been associated with more than 90% of cervical cancers in American women. It has not been proven that HPV causes the cancers, but the association between the two is definite. The virus has also been associated with cancer of the vulva in women and penile cancer in men. Babies delivered vaginally to women with genital warts may develop growths of the larynx (vocal cords) called papillomas.

The interval from infection with HPV until development of precancerous cells in women is variable. Rapid progression in a few weeks may occur, but usually the time frame is more like months or years. It is possible for one sexual exposure to stimulate change several years later. An abnormal PAP smear may be the first sign that a woman has an infection with this virus.

HPV can be treated with caustic solutions such as bichloracetic or trichloracetic acid and podophyllin. These solutions burn the warts off in most cases if done repetitively. The acid burns and may cause severe temporary pain. The warts may be removed surgically by using electrical cautery or by vaporizing them with a beam of laser light. Precancerous lesions of the cervix may be treated by freezing the cervix (cryotherapy) or by removing a portion of the cervix with a laser beam or with electric cautery.

In spite of these methods of treatment, one of the characteristics of HPV is its tendency to recur months or even years later. The recurrence may not be evident to the person and they may continue to transmit the virus sexually. HPV can be treated effectively and cancerous lesions removed, but careful follow-up with exams and PAP smears is essential.

Stuart's Ghost

Sally had biopsies of her cervix taken, and to her horror, the results confirmed invasive cancer of the cervix. She was advised by cancer specialists to have a radical hysterectomy to remove her uterus, cervix and lymph nodes. Never would she be able to have that child she so desperately wanted to love. Her surgery successfully cured her cancer, but during this same time her husband was examined and was found to be infected also.

One brief relationship at 17 had resulted in Sally's sterility and was now destabilizing her marriage. In spite of extensive counseling, Stan could not handle the fact that Sally had withheld information about her past from him before they married. At the time of her last visit with me they were separated. Sally is bitter and is having a difficult time understanding how God could love her.

Reflections and Perspectives

by Donald M. Joy

Should Sally have told Stan about Stuart and about her sexual history? If so, how, and when would it have been right?

Since marriage consists of "two becoming one," it is crucial that sexual history be laid on the table before the relationship reaches the point of no return. When I study pair bonding in humans, it becomes clear that in a healthy relationship there is a "truth threshold" just before sexual arousal dominates the attraction. When a person is engulfed in pain or abandonment or grief, as Sally was, sexual vulnerability is speeded up by disclosing the secrets to a sympathetic person.

Desmond Morris counted 12 steps in human pair bonding. Step six, I have observed, is the point at which healthy people trust each other enough that they spontaneously want to tell the secrets — now! If the relationship progresses slowly, step six naturally occurs before intimate kissing begins. But when one of the partners has been to bed in a previous relationship, the early steps are often skipped or rushed, and secrets often are never told.

I suspect that is what happened with Sally and Stan. It is likely that Sally was vulnerable and truthful with Stuart — her first sexual relationship. But the sexual shame of that misadventure sealed her secrets. She simply shifted into automatic sexual contact to try to recharge her devastated self respect without slowly telling the truth about her feelings of loss and shame.

Imagine Sally getting honest with Stan by saying something like this: "Stan, you have been so transparent with me about your problem with drugs, and I admire your integrity. But I have to tell you that although I am a Christian and I am not going to bed with you unless we marry, I got carried away with one guy. And after the relationship was over, I had some kind of infection or virus that the doctor had to treat. I'm not sure what it was, but you need to know that I may not be exactly the woman you hoped I was."

Making such an integrity statement is risky, of course. Stan may abandon her, destroying her best current dreams of life with him. But if he abandons her for this honest disclosure, this is the best time to lose him — certainly better than losing him after they marry, after he is infected and dis-covers her premarital affair through further health complications and tell-tale medical tests.

Another complication is this: Stan may pressure Sally for sexual favors to prove that she loves him as much as she loved Stuart. Jealousy is always lurking at the door when intimacy is developing. Stan's jealousy may cause him to play a deceptive trick on Sally that will kill two birds with one stone— stinging Sally with the shame of her failure while at the same time getting the sexual satisfaction he has been eager to experience with her before she is married to him. And she is vulnerable, then, now that her secret is out, to feel like trash if she doesn't cooperate with a hungry Stan — after all, he knows she is no virgin. A kind of sexual blackmail may be used against her in the wake of her courageous honesty.

Could Sally have avoided the cervical cancer, saved her uterus and been cured of HPV if she had gone to an OB-GYN specialist for an exam and PAP smear when she and Stuart broke up?

You can be sure that the doctor who removed the genital warts also did a PAP smear. It is possible to determine the specific strain of HPV which is causing the infection. Certain strains (16, 18, 31, 33, and 35) are more frequently associated with progression to dysplasia and cancer of the cervix. Sally's HPV virus was types 16 and 18 and placed her at risk for cervical cancer. If the physician knew this and the PAP smear was normal, she should have been advised to have smears at least every four months to check the speed with which the tissue might have been changing toward a cancerous state.

It is a good idea for any woman to have a complete gynecologic work-up including a PAP smear before she has genital contact with anyone. Many countries and states do not require a medical exam for disease detection before issuing a marriage license, mostly because so many people are sexually active before marriage. Concerned and thoughtful people should always get honest with a specialist and ask for a genital health check before becoming sexually intimate with another person. A normal exam without evidence of infection would provide the baseline for all future concerns. All women should have a pelvic exam and PAP smear when they are 18 years of age or when they become sexually active.

The male sex system is a closed system. A man can be a carrier of a virus or bacterium that causes him little or no trouble and shows no symptom to the naked eye. If he is carrying the HPV virus, and does not have visible warts, he still can be examined. The dilute solution of acetic acid (vinegar and water) can be placed on his genitalia and a trained professional can perform the examination with a microscope to see whether "pearly white" lesions are present. Men and women can infect their sexual partners without having any idea that they themselves are infected, since some HPV carriers have no symptoms or visible signs.

Since the woman's sexuality is an open system, anything introduced through the vaginal lips may move into the vaginal tract, through the cervical door and into the uterus, on through the fallopian tubes and into the pelvic cavity where the ovaries are suspended and the delicate ovum swim at ovulation in search of the fallopian corridor and an opportunity for conception. This open system is highly vulnerable to invasive and pervasive diseases which work quietly, internally and invisibly — often with no external symptoms. The complications, as in Sally's case, can be both life-threatening and life-altering. Here, as in most health issues, early detection greatly increases the possibilities of cure and prevention of serious consequences.

HPV is not curable, at least not at this time. We do not have "cures" for any virus. Like genital herpes and other viruses, HPV becomes a condition to deal with across the lifespan. Women carrying an aggressive strain of HPV should have a PAP smear every four or six months because a lab report will describe changes in the cells of the cervix. The diagnosis of cancer is usually made only after cells have moved through a series of changes called dysplasia, which periodic PAP smears can trace. Under regular gynecologic care, women with this diagnosis would have precancer treatments. In this early stage, the cancer can be held at bay and not become invasive.

Why was Sally so vulnerable to sex with Stuart? And how could she have prevented being so vulnerable to sex with anybody?

Young women, like young men, who suffer childhood loss of a stable and affectionate parental marriage are at risk of premature sexual contact, though it is by no means inevitable that they will become sexually active.

One of the simpler ways of describing this vulnerability is to talk about "skin hunger." When a child hits pubescence, he or she tends to recoil from parental affection and to sense that, "I have to find affirmation now from my life-long intimate partner." This starvation period tends to create an enormous hunger for skin contact, for affection, and contributes to both virginal male and virginal female vulnerability to touch, embrace, sexual arousal and intercourse. But where the mother and father are stable sources of visible affection to each other they literally trumpet the message to the kid: "Wait for the exclusive dream! It's worth it!"

A father's affirmation is crucial in convincing a young woman that a good man is somewhere out there waiting for her. The affirming father is a reminder, too, that any man who violates his daughter has to answer to him. If Sally's father had been affirming, her knowledge of her father's potential rage expressed toward Stuart would have tended to help her keep Stuart, an exploitive man, under control.

It is important, however, to see that Stuart, in the case of Sally, wasn't just anybody. Stuart had been sexually active before he took Sally to bed. A simple rule we all know, but rarely say out loud, is that people who have been to bed in one relationship will tend to go to bed in every relationship after that one. And we know, too, that the appetite for getting sex, once awakened, never goes away. There may be wonderful exceptions to these "rules," but they are very rare.

So if Sally had determined not to go to bed with Stan and any guys between Stuart and her future husband, she would have broken cultural patterns in dating. Because of her increased vulnerability, after Stuart she would need to keep future relationships "in public" and to avoid complete privacy with the guy at all costs.

Would you say Sally is an immoral person because she had sex with Stuart? Isn't morality a matter of religious belief?

Anything is moral, universally, if it holds potential for enhancing the quality of human life. All really comprehensive religious systems pay attention to "moral issues" because religion, by definition, is always targeted on enhancing the quality of human life. But religions do not invent morality. So when we look at the many questions women and men ask about the issues raised by Dr. Hager's case studies, there is always a moral dimension.

Some people naively think that religious people think that sex is immoral, but deeply religious people know that human sexuality is the gift of the "image of

God." Sex offers the highest rewards available: two-become-one intimacy, parenthood and life-long enhancement of self respect. Because of sex, human beings can have the satisfaction of growing old, wise and full of years and celebrating the birth, growth and launching of grandchildren. I can testify that it doesn't get any better than that! And because human sexuality is "standard equipment on all models," everyone has an opportunity for these grand blessings.

But when human sexuality is handled carelessly it is the source of the greatest human tragedy, pain and disaster. Few griefs are more tragic than those you will read about in Dr. Hager's casebook.

It is easy to become a sexual victim. Since our sexuality is at the core of our personhood, we are vulnerable to sexual violence,

exploitation and bankruptcy. The word "rape" speaks of sexual exploitation, but we also speak of being "raped" as we refer to virtually every kind of violent rip-off humans experience: financial, professional, work-related, even wrong-headed religious advice and treatment. This illustrates that sexual vulnerability can lead to the ultimate personal loss. Almost everything about our sexuality is wrapped in moral consequences: our pleasure, our fertility, our identity and our sense of self respect.

I could send you to the Judeo-Christian textbook — the Old Testament and the New Testament which Christians combine to call the Holy Bible. The Bible contains sexual cases, laws and consequences for "fornication" (promiscuity and sexual addiction), for adultery (carrying the ghost of a past relationship into a new one), for rape, for incest and for homosexual activity. But in every case, the rule and the consequences consistently express God's commitment to the highest quality of life for humans.

In looking at Dr. Hager's cases in this book, we will pay attention to the deep moral question. We can be sure that the only solutions — whether they are cures, treatment or altered values and life-style, or all of these — are explicitly addressed in the Bible and are consistent with the highest Judeo-Christian vision of what humans are and what they are capable of becoming.

St. Paul warns us not to "wrong or exploit a brother or a sister in this matter, because the Lord is an avenger in all these things." And "these things" have to do with your "sanctification: that you abstain from fornication; that each one of you know how to control your own body in holiness and honor, not with lustful passion like the Gentiles who do not know God" (1 Thessalonians 4:3-6 NRSV). Link these warnings with the Old Testament commandments about telling the truth and exclusive sexual fidelity in marriage, and you have the Judeo-Christian bottom line. But the Apostle Paul and the Jewish Ten Commandments did not invent sexual morality. They only remind us of natural consequences and put sexuality in a universal perspective as urgently demanding honesty in relationships.

In this chapter Sally's case identifies urgent issues for any woman. These include problems associated with having sexual contact with a man with previous sexual experience, and with acquiring external symptoms that can be removed without revealing a more serious internal disease at work. Sally's case also demonstrates the difficulty of maintaining the persistent vision of a monogamous and abundantly rich marriage and family life while dealing with the conse-quences of early vulnerability in the arms of her first, and what she thought would be her only, love. As we have seen, the basic policy of transparent honesty is a way to move with integrity from loss or failure.

Chapter Two

A Double-Edged Sword

by W. David Hager, M.D.

One night after a lengthy high school football practice, several of my friends and I decided to climb a sheer cliff to a campsite above, instead of taking the long way around by a dirt road. We struggled and slipped and clawed our way to the top in the darkness, never pausing to think that we could tumble to our deaths in the falls many feet below us.

On another exciting evening when I was in high school, three of my best friends and I decided to drive our car down a two-lane highway with the lights off just for the thrill of it. We felt immortal, and never considered that we might hurt someone else.

My best friend, Steve, once gave me a machete that he had obtained in Zaire, Africa where his parents were missionaries. The beautiful weapon had a hand-carved handle and gleaming double-edged blade. When pulled from its sheath, it could easily slash its owner if he or she did not remove it carefully. I still have a scar on my right hand from that machete.

These tales from my youth illustrate the way it is

31

when we play around sexually. In spite of all that we
know, we feel that we are untouchable, that nothing can
hurt us. We grasp that double-edged sword, taking
something which really is not ours, just for the immediate pleasure. We end up wounding ourselves, and others.
Nan's story is about one of those double-edged risks.

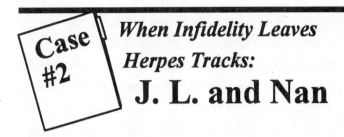

Case #2
When Infidelity Leaves Herpes Tracks:
J. L. and Nan

Nan is a twenty-one-year-old, single woman who grew up in a devout Christian home with godly parents. She had dated a great deal in high school and college before meeting J. L. He was a campus leader, majoring in political science and intending to enter law school. The couple dated extensively and fell in love.

From the beginning of the relationship, J. L. tried to convince Nan to have sexual intercourse. She refused time after time. She did not feel this was reason enough to stop the relationship, even though she felt that from a moral and spiritual perspective premarital intercourse was wrong.

'You Are My First Love'

One evening, on the anniversary of their first meeting, J. L. finally convinced Nan to celebrate their year by having their first intercourse. J. L. had told her repeatedly that he had never before been sexually active. He had, however, actually engaged in intercourse with two other women. He had contracted herpes genital infection from one of these encounters, but after an initial episode with genital blisters, J. L.'s symptoms had never recurred. He did not know what the blisters were and was unaware that he was carrying the disease.

Nan made an appointment to see me for a pre-marital examination, one month prior to her wedding. The day before her appointment, she began experiencing severe itching and pain of the outside of the vagina — the vulva. She was found to have multiple blisters and ulcerative sores on the vulva. The diagnosis was immediately apparent. She was devastated when I informed her that she had a sexually transmitted disease caused by a virus that is spread by intimate contact. Her disease, I told her, is called herpes genital infection.

Herpes Simplex — HSV

The virus is named Herpes simplex (HSV). There are two principal types: I and II. Type I causes most oral-labial herpes — fever blisters on the mouth, or cold sores. Type II causes most genital herpes, although either type can cause the opposite infections as a result of oral-genital contact. Previous exposure to Type I HSV may decrease the severity of a Type II outbreak, but it does not prevent disease.

Shaken Relationship

Nan resolved her infection very slowly over the next three weeks, but her emotional wounds were much slower to heal. She talked with J. L., broke the engagement and cancelled the wedding. They have recently begun to date again. She has had numerous recurrences of herpes blisters and has begun medication using acyclovir suppression. She has responded with a marked decrease in recurrences and is learning to cope with her disease.

How Herpes Is Transmitted

An estimated 400,000 new cases of HSV are diagnosed in the United States each year. Many persons who are infected never manifest symptoms and thus are unaware that they harbor the virus. Some researchers have estimated that up to 60% of the adult population in the U.S. has been infected with the virus.

HSV is transmitted by direct intimate contact between individuals. Although transmission by towels, clothing, toilet seats and such has been suggested, this occurs rarely, if ever. The virus normally infects mucosal surfaces such as the inside of the vagina or the inside of the mouth or the lips. The virus can also enter the skin at sites of cuts or abrasions. This is frequently the way in which infection occurs — at points irritated by intercourse. HSV may cause an initial infection and then migrate to sites beneath the skin on nerve cells. From these nerves, the organism may later return to the surface to cause recurrences of infection.

HSV Symptoms

It takes five to seven days from the time of initial exposure to HSV before evidence of infection occurs. The symptoms of infection are tingling, itching and burning at the site where lesions will develop. The virus causes small raised bumps called papules which then become fluid-filled blisters — vesicles. These blisters then break down into raw sores called ulcers which are usually very painful. In addition to pain, the infected person may have swollen lymph nodes, muscle aches and difficulty urinating.

One of the major problems in dealing with HSV is that many persons will not have any symptoms from their infection. Some investigators have found only 25 to 50% of persons with documented infection show symptoms. Regardless of whether the initial infection caused symptoms, 60 to 70% of patients will have recurrences of HSV. Usually, the recurrences are not as severe as the initial symptomatic episode. In addition to chronic recurrences causing symptoms, the patient frequently experiences depression and interference with sexual intimacy.

Herpes Treatment

Acyclovir is an antiviral medication that can be administered orally or used as a topical cream applied directly to the HSV symptom blisters. With an acute symptomatic outbreak, the treatment consists of five 200 mg. capsules daily for five days. For persons with frequent recurrences we use two to three 200 mg. capsules daily for six to nine months continuously. The frequency of recurrences can be reduced by 40 to 80%. In relationships where only one person is infected, condoms should be used to try to decrease the chance of spreading the virus to another person.

Herpes and Newborns

Babies can be infected with HSV. Most of these infections occur when the baby passes through the cervix and vagina, but the virus can be spread through the placenta directly to the baby during pregnancy. There are 350 to 400 cases of neonatal HSV each year in the United States. Most of the mothers whose babies are infected had no idea that they were infected. Of those babies who develop HSV, the mortality rate has been reported to be 70%. And of those who survive, 83% have learning disorders. Acyclovir may have some effect on these ominous statistics. If a mother avoids a recurrent outbreak of herpes at the time of delivery, the chance of transmission to the baby is much less, occurring only 5 to 8% of the time.

Reflections and Perspectives

by Donald M. Joy

Why did J. L. lie to Nan saying he had never been sexually active? Could he have meant that he had never been married or had a long-term sexual relationship? What good is pledging that we are literally "virgins" or "not virgins" if he can weasel out of the truth like that?

Most people do not tell the truth early in a relationship. When asked about past relationships, our first instinct is to protect ourselves. We translate the probe as, "Are you a good and safe person for me?" So that is the question we tend to answer.

If we give J. L. the benefit of that doubt, then we assume he was eager to put the two brief sexual encounters behind him. He likely was sorry to have had sexual intercourse with those two women, so he brushed them aside. After all, he may have reasoned, "I got my punishment! I remember those awful sores I had after that one time! I'm relieved that God warned me, so I repented. If God forgave me, then the past doesn't count."

On the other hand, in a worst case scenario, J. L. was an outright liar. He told Nan what he knew would break down her virginal resistance to him. The oldest con game of all sexual seductions is: "I've never loved anyone like I love you."

So it is just this simple. Men and women considering marriage need to haul their partners off to the physician for a complete STD analysis before the genitals touch. Yet even this is not totally preventive. The antiquated blood test once required in almost every state in the United States is obviously too unsophisticated for today's parade of terrifying and sometimes deadly diseases.

Can Nan and J. L. ever make marriage work?

We hope so. In a sense, they were both naive. J. L. lied and seduced her, then infected her for a lifetime. Everything depends on how he shoulders final responsibility for that sequence of crimes against Nan. The marriage will not work if Nan cannot find peace with the infecting episode. She may successfully eliminate most symptoms most of the time, but her emotions and her affections will be toxic if J. L.'s violation of her and her health is not resolved through J. L.'s emotional and spiritual restitution. He must pay her back through repentance and commitment to life-long responsibility, fidelity and care. There is time in an orderly dating relationship for her to determine whether this man has integrity or not. The seduction episode says a loud NO to that issue. A long-term dating exploration, however, may eventually erase that assault on honesty and care.

How can Nan ever forgive J. L.? Really, because of him her whole life has been changed forever.

Forgiveness is a choice, so this question is crucial to both Nan and J. L. for the remainder of their lives.

Sometimes, especially when teaching our children, we demand instant forgiveness: Say, "I'm sorry!" Now, say, "I forgive you!" Quick forgiveness almost always leads to a thinly covered resentment that will simmer as long as memory lasts. Quick forgiveness is another form of denial, of lying in order to "be a good person." Here are some tips for Nan, should she want to travel the road to emotional and spiritual healing, regardless of what happens to their relationship:

1. **Forgiveness first re-quires "counting the losses."** This means that Nan must face the truth about what happened, and must sort out "who did what to whom" and "with what motives." This will give Nan a clearer sense of what part she played in the sexual activity that transmitted the herpes virus. She will be able to grieve over J. L.'s lying, over his pressuring her to have intercourse and over his failure to even take care of his own genital infection which had shown up after one of his earlier sexual partnerships.

"Getting the facts straight" is an essential first step in deciding whether to forgive.

2. **Nan needs to grieve.** And she must do this alone. People who can walk through her memory of the "facts" can "weep with her" as Jesus urged. But the grief work is Nan's lonely work — going "through the valley of the shadow of death." When Nan has counted the losses and has started her long grief process, she may be ready to make the forgiveness decision.

3. **True Forgiveness means "choosing to pay twice."** When anyone forgives — whether a debt, an act of violence, a sexual virus — that person deliberately chooses to

"commute" the perpetrator's crime. When "commutation" occurs, the guilt shifts from the criminal to the one who hs been violated. Nan must be able to say, "J. L. I forgive you. What you did to me, I take as if *I* were the one who lied, who pressured and who hid the history of genital blisters. Whenever I think of what has happened, I will blame myself, not you."

Only when the full load of responsibility shifts to the person forgiving can Nan's emotional and spiritual center relax and be at peace. Jesus, on the cross, took the sins of others as his own as he taught us what it is to forgive: "Father, forgive them. They do not know what they are doing."

We hope that Nan can forgive J. L. The second phase may be even harder for each of them: forgiving themselves for what they messed up and damaged permanently, for reducing their relationship to sex. The viral disease is a reminder that the best and most beautiful intimacy for which they were created has been forever marred with disease. The same grief process, which takes time, is urgent work for each of them, as they make peace with themselves. If they cannot forgive themselves, they will not be able to live with each other.

Is exclusive sex — one guy and one woman — possible today?

Let's examine both answers — "Yes" and "No" — and follow them to some conclusions. Then, decide for yourself.

Yes. A universal "dream" of every boy and

girl is that somewhere exists one exclusive, life-long intimate partner. This is true regardless of religious tradition and ethnic origin. Only children whose sexual boundaries have been violated by seduction or molestation seem to have no "ultimate private citadel" dream of an exclusive monogamous union.

More than 50 years ago, J. D. Unwin found that the only Stone Age cultures to thrive had three characteristics:

1. They protected the sexual integrity of their children and prevented pre-marriage sexual contact.
2. They limited marriage to one man and one woman and forbade sexual activity outside of marriage.
3. They practiced worship of one God who was honored by building a shrine with a roof tall enough to enter and stand while performing worship rituals.

Unwin found, too, that only those cultures which consistently held all three values were vital cultures. He described their strengths as (a) cultural vitality — a high energy level in production and providing for everyone's needs; (b) cultural creativity — inventiveness and progressive modernization; and (c) cultural expansiveness — they carved out more land and resources from untamed territories and actually planted their own people in this new space.

So, we can say, "Yes, exclusive, lifelong monogamy is both possible and desirable." But it is not an easy or natural path. The natural way is the lazy way — indifferent child rearing, carelessly living out a marriage and idolatry in religion in which we worship anything which catches our fancy. When we do not build significant temples and practice intentional worship which has a transcendent quality to it, there is no openness to the skies!

No. Now try the answer "No." If we decide that "one man – one woman" relationships are impossible today, it will be because we choose to go with the flow of popular culture. We have a strong need to feel that we are "approved" by our friends. If approval means getting sex early and with many partners, then we will likely squelch our private vision of exclusive and lifelong loving and go for social status. To complicate all of this, our culture daily bombards us with messages which portray promiscuity as "normal." These range from music lyrics and explicit movies to promotion of school-based condom dispensaries to distorted statistics which promote as "fact" that more than half of our teenagers are "sexually active." (Both secular and religious statistics are doubled and sometimes tripled to make the point. Secular distortions obviously aim to create sensational headlines while softening up the virginal vision of the young. Religious distortions seek to use fear to stir families to better parental supervision. Not surprisingly, both distortions lead to increased sexual activity because of the social pressure they create.)

So, with such pressures on our young and our single adults, it is easy for us to cave in and say, "No, the one man and one woman vision is not possible today."

Even so, the amazing good news is this: Many people love each other so much that they painfully and intentionally "make it to the church on time" and limit their sexual contact to one exclusive partner. And others who have had a sexual misadventure manage to come home to integrity and find themselves transformed and ready to live out the exclusive dream with a person to whom they have disclosed the whole truth.

J. L. and Nan's story reminds us of the urgent need to be honest and postpone sexual contact until a complete medical exam clears the way for marriage and exclusive sex. J. L.'s mildly promiscuous but hidden past re-opens the perennial question about premarital sex. His sexual demands on Nan remind us that the popular idea in our culture is that getting sex is a person's right, that waiting is for people who aren't winners. A common attitude is, "I want what I want when I want it, and that's the test of your love for me!"

What becomes clearer with every case from Dr. Hager's files is that God's way of exclusively monogamous sexual intimacy is the medical, moral and emotional path to peace and health. Profound intimacy results from gentle, respect-based love that protects the future before consummating in the ultimate intercourse.

Chapter Three

An Emergency in the Sky

by W. David Hager, M.D.

Recently I took a transcontinental flight to Seattle, Washington. Midway across the country, a flight attendant suddenly interrupted the silence of the moment with a plea, "If there is a doctor on board please come to Row 17, Seat C immediately." I looked around for another physician to bolt to the scene, but no one moved.

I hurried to 17C to find a panic stricken 14-year-old girl, pupils dilated, frantically griping the arms of her seat and gasping for breath. She was having an acute asthmatic attack with a constricting spasm of her airway resulting in wheezing and shortness of breath. Fortunately, the flight had a well equipped emergency kit, and I was able to administer medication to get her out of bronchospasm and back to normal breathing.

I was puzzled about why she had such a severe attack out of the blue, or should I say in the blue. She explained that she has severe allergies to foods, including nuts. There were minced nuts in the plum sauce that covered the chicken served for lunch on the flight. The nuts were chopped so small that I hadn't even noticed them. The girl said, "I never would have eaten the food if I had known there were nuts in there." As I reflected on the girl's failure to request a "nut free" meal, I realized that her lack of communication had nearly resulted in a tragedy.

In our relationships with others, communication and understanding are keys to love and intimacy. We need a certain amount of knowledge about each other in order to meet each others' needs. If we are committed to this type of communication, we will often find the capacity to help heal each others' past pain and move into a new realm of togetherness, self-respect and high regard for each other. The story of Tammie and Robert illustrates what can happen when we fail to communicate honestly.

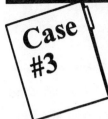

Case #3

Self-Pity, Street Sex and Telltale Gonorrhea

Tammie's Story

Tammie is a 32-year-old mother of one child. Her husband is a minister. She was reared in a very conservative home by her mother and her stepfather. He had abused Tammie sexually when she was between the ages of 9 and 12. She had succeeded in burying those memories of abuse, denying they had ever happened.

Tammie dated Robert off and on during their college years and married him during their senior year. After graduation, she worked as a secretary to help put Robert through graduate school.

As a result of the traumatic events of her childhood, Tammie had great difficulty with sexual intimacy. She loved Robert but could not express her feelings to him and frequently chose to avoid sexual intercourse. In spite of infrequent contact, she conceived and they had a son during his second year in seminary.

Robert's Self Pity

Tammie became suspicious that her husband was frequenting houses of prostitution when she unexpectedly saw him entering such an establishment in a nearby town one night. She followed him on another occasion and saw the event repeat itself. She was panic-stricken, but dared not confront Robert for fear that he would lash out about her frigidity. She remembered how she had been told by her step-father never to reveal his sexual contact with her.

I saw her in the office shortly thereafter with a complaint of a yellow vaginal discharge. She had no other symptoms and insisted that her husband had no complaints of burning with urination or discharge from the penis. A culture of the discharge grew *Neisseria gonorrheae*, the bacterium that causes gonorrhea, known on the street as "the clap." She was treated with an injectable antibiotic and with seven days of oral tetracycline. She responded readily to the treatment and her discharge ceased. The follow-up culture was negative.

Robert became irate and very defensive when confronted with the information that his wife had gonorrhea. He accused her of having gone out on him and said that she was a disgrace to his future ministry. After a long conference with the couple, he reluctantly confessed his unfaithfulness, agreed to being treated with an antibiotic and consented to counseling.

I asked Robert if he had ever stopped to consider the consequences of his behavior.

"No," he responded, "I felt that Tammie was unreasonably aloof and frigid, and I had to have a sexual outlet. I couldn't talk to her about it. I thought prostitutes took antibiotics to prevent infections, and I never thought I would get a sexually transmitted disease anyway. If I had known about the consequences, I never would have done this."

Gonorrhea — 'The Clap'

Gonorrhea (GC) is caused by a bacterium named *Neisseria gonorrheae* or the gonococcus. One million cases of gonorrhea are reported each year through public health services in the U. S. Since many cases are not reported, it is estimated that two million new cases actually occur each year. When a woman has intercourse with a male infected with GC, she has a 40% chance of becoming infected. It takes three to five days from the time of exposure for symptoms to develop.

When gonorrhea is present, the symptoms, if any, will show up in the lower genital tract: the urethra and rectum in men, the vagina, cervix, urethra and rectum in women. The symptoms tend to show up in men as abnormal discharge from the penis and burning upon urination. In women there maybe an abnormal discharge from the vagina. It is common, as with chlamydial infections, for a person to harbor the organism and yet show no symptoms at all. All the same, the person with no symptoms may infect his or her partners.

Studies on this infection indicate that 80% of all women infected will not have symptoms. Men more frequently show symptoms with gonorrhea. A known fact is that STDs often occur together. For example, 30% of women with gonorrhea will have a chlamydial infection as well.

The gonococcus can ascend through the cervix and uterus in women and infect the fallopian tubes. Once infected, the tubes, which transport ova (eggs) from the ovaries to the uterus, may become swollen and blocked off. This blockage can result in infertility, chronic pain and tubal (ectopic) pregnancy. Partially due to the high rates of chlamydia and gonorrhea, there is an "epidemic" of infertility and tubal pregnancy in this country. Fifteen to eighteen percent of all marriages are complicated by infertility. The incidence of tubal pregnancy is rising annually in the U.S. In addition to resulting in fetal loss it can cause maternal death.

Recovery

Fortunately, *Neisseria gonorrheae* can be killed by tetracycline antibiotics such as doxycycline given in a dose of 100 mg. twice a day for seven days. Newer strains of the organism have developed resistance to penicillins and pose a threat to our management of gonorrhea infections. At present, these strains can be treated with certain cephalosporin antibiotics such as rocephin 250 mg. in an injection. Not only must both sexual partners be treated, but any other partners they have had recently must also take antibiotics in order to prevent further spread of the disease.

Prognosis?

Tammie and Robert are in therapy for their phobias and addictions. Robert has come to understand the reasons behind Tammie's fear of sexual intimacy. Tammie understands Robert's tendency to seek compensatory sexual satisfaction and his vulnerability to becoming sexually addicted to intercourse for its own sake. He has recognized his capacity for sin. Together they have claimed Colossians 2:8 as their scripture verse: "See to it that no one takes you captive through hollow and deceptive philosophy, which depends on human tradition and the basic principles of this world rather than on Christ."

Reflections and Perspectives

by Donald M. Joy

Why is early sexual abuse so devastating to a woman?

Sexual exploration among children of the same age and inexperience rarely leaves scars in adult life. Indeed, unless such "sex play" or exploration is interrupted with an emotionally charged adult reaction, it is rarely remembered. Sex play is a way of finding out how the world works.

But when an adult or older child takes the initiative with a child, the effects are virtually permanent. The victim is almost always inappropriately fascinated with sexuality. They tend to see themselves as "a sex object — nothing more!" Devastated self-respect is a core response, though this is often missed when the person is so "sexually active." We assume that a pro-miscuous person, for example, has no problem with self esteem. Among women especially, the adult response is to opt out of sexual intimacy, to freeze up. "I do not feel like a wife, a woman, or a mother," one sexually inhibited woman confessed.

Both women and men show long-term effects of early adult initiated sexual seduction. Men are more likely to split their search for sexual pleasure from their sense of self and their career. The clandestine rapist, voyeur, exposer, womanizer, homosexual and pornography addict very often was used early in life for sexual purposes.

The male reproductive sex system is essentially a pleasure system. With normal hormonal production, men, in general, tend to pursue a high frequency outlet. With the mid-life hormonal waning, many men become emotionally more alive and less sexually driven. This often means that older men require the same emotional care that women need if they are to be sexually competent. And since penetration is impossible with the slightest emotional wavering, male dysfunction is easier to identify than that of the female who can continue to "go through the motions" even while devastated emotionally.

The female reproductive sex system, in contrast, works like clockwork, with pleasure separated from fertility. The ovulation cycle works without stimulation or pleasure, creating no urgent physiological sense of "need" for fertility release. Among women, therefore, it is common to find many victims of sexual abuse or emotional trauma who have simply withered at the core of their personhood. They withdraw from vulnerability and intimacy which require trust and bring the potential for another violation.

There is good evidence, too, that women are more organized around emotional sensitivity than men. They are more likely to pay attention to their own feelings and are more aware of other people's emotional states than men. This means that for many women the scene must be just right if they are to respond sexually. Like the sensitive plant which closes its leaves when touched, a woman may shut down emotionally and sexually at the slightest reminder of her past pain or her present perceived worthlessness.

How does incest happen? Especially between a parent and a child?

Incest happens when

some well-defined universal boundaries break down. All humans crave privacy and tend to grant privacy to others. Parental affection for children, indeed all adult affection for children, is normally based on respect and anticipation of a good future for the children. It is a universal happy condition when adults know their children are sexual beings who will establish sexual relationships with appropriate exclusive partners when marriage occurs. Healthy adults assist children in reaching that peak experience of marriage and sexual union by using elaborate rituals of encouraging social contact (such as dating) and throwing a grand celebration (such as a wedding) to give public and visible recognition to the private and sacred mystery of sexual intimacy.

Anything which breaks down these boundaries of privacy, respect and antici-pated celebration of sexual fulfillment can set the stage for adult-child incest. The common boundary smashers are:

1. The adult was abused as a child, so assumes sexual "use" is normal. In any case, the abuse is a way of retaliating against what was done in the adult's childhood.

2. The adult has — due to past abuse or other reasons — lost self-respect. No one can respect other people if his or her self-respect is low. "Love your neighbor as you love yourself" could be bad advice for a person who has no self-respect.

3. Multiple sexual partners at any time in life tends to break down the boundary that protects anyone from becoming the next partner.

When a step-father initiates sexual activity with a step-daughter, we might see all three factors at work. This may be a second or third marriage for the step-father. The daughter came with the territory of the new marriage, and as she blossoms or as he anticipates that she is about to turn into a ripened woman, she becomes his next target.

This sexual targeting tends to occur at a higher rate in step-families than in first marriage families. Boundaries between blended family siblings also seem to be fragile. The simple axiom at work among socially available potential partners seems to work in the blended families: Time spent together lowers boundaries and favors sexual bonding or sexual exploitation. Therefore, it is important to create a respect-based environment in the home and in social settings.

What makes people think they can be promiscuous without being caught by disease and other consequences? I cannot believe Robert's statement that he never thought he would contract a sexually transmitted disease when he was using prostitutes!

We are all born with an invincible will to live, to survive. Because of this, we imagine that what happens to other people will never happen to us. Jean Piaget called it, unfortunately, "egocentrism." We misunderstand this term to mean egomania — the idea that what I want is the only important thing in the world. But Piaget was simply describing this central tendency of humans — especially children and teens — to see everything but themselves. We stand outside the objective world and watch disaster, but cannot imagine that we are part of that world and potential victims of the same disaster.

Unfortunately, many adults continue to believe that they are outside the normal world of other folks — that bad things may happen to others, but not to them. Oddly enough, this is similar to a very popular Christian cultic view. "I thought I was special to God," one 23-year old woman told me, "but he let me down and let me get pregnant. Always before when my boyfriend and I had sinned and repented, I never got pregnant." The idea that being religious immunizes a person from trouble is only a spiritual version of this naive egocentrism.

Why didn't Robert pay attention to Tammie's real problem instead of going outside the marriage to get his own sexual pleasure?

It is clear that Tammie and Robert were both consumed by their own needs and had not reached the point in their marriage of meeting each other's needs. Counselors commonly hear blame statements, "It's her problem!" or, "It's his problem!" Instead, anything that affects either partner is "our problem." The Judeo-Christian concept of "two becoming one" in marriage is a mystery, but it works only when each person makes the other's well-being a priority. Conselors also frequently hear, "I wouldn't be the way I am if he or she wasn't the way they are" or, "If that person wouldn't do to me what he or she is doing, I'd be different." But no recovery begins until a person sorts out responsibility "facts" without blaming anyone. The healing journey begins with a first step of "owning my part of the problem" and releasing other people to their own journeys of recovery and making their own painful confessions of failure and responsibility.

When this "two caring persons as one" occurs, they read each others' words, faces and body language and turn all of the messages into constructive action. This martial communication is often painful, but it is essential to developing a mature and strong marriage and the basis for a healthy family.

Robert was really behaving like a wounded little boy who had to look out for his own needs. Self-pity leads quickly and inevitably to destructive behavior. You can justify anything, literally *anything*, if you feel sorry enough for yourself. You can do compensatory sex and justify it on the basis of your need for intimacy. You can abuse, abandon or even murder to "get even" with

someone because you were hurt or neglected.

Two cures for Robert's attraction for promiscuous and prostituted sex are to

1. Establish a high-communication, high-respect, "I-am-my-spouse's caregiver!" marriage.
2. Ground himself in healthy self-esteem.

Christians commitment calls us to "come and die," to sacrifice all and to follow Jesus, and provides a high sense of self-value. "Being" becomes more important than "doing," especially than "doing sex" for compensatory reasons. The paradox is that in giving up we gain; in dying to self, we are able to find life in all of its fullness.

In this chapter we have looked at a sexual abuse victim's troubled marriage which was complicated by prostitution and gonorrhea.

We have traced a common cluster of problems ranging from the removal of boundaries which prevent parent-child incest to the role of self-pity in motivating compensatory sexual activity outside of the marriage.

While the physiological problems of STDs are the driving plot line of this book, it is clear that healthy personhood and high-respect, high-communication marriages can set the stage for prevention of STDs. High-regard marriages provide enormous emotional, spiritual and physiological protection.

Chapter Four

One Hot Summer Night

by W. David Hager, M.D.

It was a hot summer night in the small town where I
grew up. I recall the rising clamor of the large crowd in
the high school gymnasium, the smell of cigarette smoke
in the air and the moisture of the sweaty arms of tall men
rubbing against my shirt as they walked past. I certainly
was glad that my small pre-adolescent hand was encased
in the grip of my father's strong left hand. He led me to
a bleacher seat and left me with a friend while he proceeded to the platform amid taunts and jeers. "Go to
hell, Hager! You nigger lover!" someone yelled. I was
frozen to my seat, immobile with fear.

My father was superintendent of the county's school
system. It was a time of great racial unrest in the South.
Names like Martin Luther King, Medger Evers and
Ralph Abernathy were in the headlines. Dad had made
the decision that it was time to integrate the county's
schools. Many long, tumultuous meetings had taken
place. Ugly words, taunts and threats had been spoken,
but finally the school board had agreed with his convic-
tion and a resolution was passed. The county's ministe-

rial association was canvassed and had agreed by a small
margin to support the resolution. They had promised to
be present the night of the meeting in the school gym,
but not one pastor showed up.

The meeting was being held to announce the decision
to the residents of the community. The word had leaked
out, however, and people had come to voice their dis-
pleasure. "White man's traitor," someone screamed as
Dad began to speak. How he was able to get through the
announcement amazed me. His calm, strong voice
seemed to mellow even the most vociferous dissident.
Until I found my first-born son lying on the bottom of a
swimming pool and rescued him by desperate resuscitation, I would never be as scared as I was that night.

The mob's actions did not stop with shouting words.
My father was hung in effigy later that week and a cross
was burned one night on our front lawn. I learned a lot
about forgiveness in many talks I had with my Dad after
that event, but the feeling of being violated and abandoned by friends is a painful memory. The courage that I
witnessed in my mother's and father's lives and the
effects that sin had on innocent lives in those days were
resurrected in my mind when I heard Brenda's story in
my office.

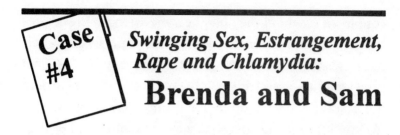

Swinging Sex, Estrangement, Rape and Chlamydia:

Brenda and Sam

Brenda was a 26-year-old mother of a young child. The product of a broken home, her father had abandoned the family when she was 10 years old. Brenda was devastated by her parents' divorce and felt betrayed by the father she had loved.

She fell in love with the first boy her mother allowed her to date. He was four years older than Brenda and convinced her to marry him when she graduated from high school. A pregnancy soon followed.

Though Brenda was a very young wife and mother, she was determined to bring certain standards to her home. Early in her life, she had accepted Christ during a revival in her local church. It seemed only natural to her to take her small daughter to church. Her husband, Sam, had no such beliefs or standards, and did not support her efforts to make her personal relationship with Christ a part of their marriage and home.

Sam Demands Group Sex

Buried deep within Sam's subconscious mind was the memory of early sexual abuse. Now an adult, the effects of this abuse manifested themselves in Sam's and Brenda's sex life. To Brenda's horror, her husband began to suggest that they participate in group sex with a couple with whom they had become friends. Brenda resisted, but Sam became more and more persistent. Their marriage teetered on the brink of destruction as Sam threatened to desert his small family if his wife would not comply with his desires and play his sexual games. Young, jobless and completely dependent upon her husband, Brenda finally relented.

Once the deed was done, she was sickened at the realization of what she had agreed to do. Brenda told Sam that she would never participate in these "games" again. True to his word, Sam moved out. His life turned from bad to worse as his life-style became more and more decadent and his drinking increased. Ultimately he lost his job and returned to Brenda begging for another chance to be a family. Because of her commitment to Christ and her marriage vows, Brenda felt compelled to take her husband back, even though her feelings of disgust and betrayal had not abated.

Marital Rape and an STD

Sam came home but it wasn't long before a pattern of verbal abuse began to emerge. Once again, she refused to be sexually intimate with him unless his behavior changed. Angrily, he spurned all of her attempts to talk and reason together and was adamantly opposed to any outside help in the form of counseling. Verbal abuse gave way to physical abuse and one hot summer night, the violence escalated when Sam forcibly raped his wife.

This time the marriage ended for good but not without consequences to Brenda. A few months after the rape, blood tests confirmed that she was pregnant. Hidden from Brenda was the fact that she had been infected by a sexually transmitted bacterium, Chlamydia trachomatis, at the same time that she had become pregnant. Because of her embarrassment about the events surrounding the conception and Sam's absence from the home, Brenda did not seek medical care until late in her pregnancy.

In another physician's office, she was examined and found to be 26 weeks (6 months) pregnant. She had no symptoms of infection, and no cultures were done. She had complaints of lower abdominal pain but no cause could be found.

I saw Brenda for the first time at 27.5 weeks gestation when she presented herself at the hospital, eight centimeters dilated, in preterm labor. Her contractions could not be stopped, and shortly after arriving on the labor and delivery unit she delivered a two-pound, preterm infant. The baby died the following day of severe hyaline membrane disease, a condition in premature infants where the lungs cannot remain expanded to contain oxygen. The baby was infected with chlamydia and cultures from Brenda's cervix were also positive for chlamydia.

Chlamydia

Chlamydia is one of the most frequent STDs in the United States with more than three million new cases estimated annually. It is also the leading infectious cause of blindness in the world. Particular infections caused by this organism include those of the urethra, epididymis, prostate and rectum in men. In women the infections attack the urethra, cervix, uterus, fallopian tubes, lymph nodes in the groin and the outside of the liver. The lungs and eyes in newborn babies can be infected at birth from passage through their mother's birth canal.

Studies indicate that 30-35% of all patients seen in STD clinics have chlamydia. An astonishing figure is that 10-18% of women in college are reported to have been infected with this organism. Since STDs often occur together, many of these young women may have another infection as well.

The time from infection until symptoms develop may vary from a few days to two weeks. The initial effects of infection may be minimal, allowing significant damage to occur before the patient seeks medical care. Current information indicates that 60-80% of women who are infected have no symptoms at all.

Women who are infected may have a heavy, yellowish vaginal discharge, if they have any symptoms at all. Because this bacterium attaches to columnar epithelial cells — cells that line the inside of the cervix and uterus — and not squamous cells — cells that line the inside of the vagina — it does not cause vaginitis in adults. Infection of the cervix may spread into the uterus and out to the fallopian tubes causing pain in the pelvis and abdomen.

Men are more often symptomatic than women. Frequent symptoms in males are discharge from the penis and burning with urination. Men without symptoms may transmit the organism without knowing that they are infected.

Damage, Diagnosis and Treatment

Chlamydia infections can be diagnosed by taking a culture from the area of infection or by using special fluorescent stains on the discharge to allow identification of chlamydia antibodies under the microscope. *Chlamydia traehomatis* responds to antibiotic treatment in most situations of localized infection. However, when the infection has spread control may be difficult. Tetracycline, 500 mg. four times daily for seven days, or doxycycline, 100 mg. twice daily for seven days, are the antibiotics of choice for treatment. Some recent evidence indicates that ampicillin may have some beneficial effect in treating chlamydia. Erythromycin, 500 mg. four times daily for seven days, is used to treat chlamydia in pregnancy where tetracycline cannot be used because of the risk of staining the baby's teeth or affecting the baby's bones.

If the infection spreads to the fallopian tubes in women, it can cause an infection called pelvic inflammatory disease (PID). More than one million cases of PID are reported in the United States annually. Unfortunately, this infection can result in serious damage to the tubes before the patient develops symptoms that normally alert her to seek medical care. The fallopian tubes are lined by small hair-like structures called cilia. The cilia act to propel an egg from the ovary to the uterus. When chlamydiae infect the tubes, they shear off the cilia at their base and cause the inside surface to be barren, thereby more likely to be infected and less likely to be able to move a fertilized egg through the tube to its site of implantation in the uterus. The term "a barren woman" takes on greater significance when you have seen tubes damaged in this way.

Women with PID may have fever, chills, abnormal vaginal discharge and abdominal pain. However, many have no symptoms until the disease has progressed to the point of tubal damage.

I have published a paper on the criteria for the diagnosis of this disorder, but regret having to report that even experienced doctors make an incorrect diagnosis of PID more than 35% of the time. Delays in diagnosis can result in irreparable damage to the fallopian tubes. Tubal damage can then result in infertility, ectopic (tubal) pregnancies or chronic pain.

PID is treated with antibiotics. We treat many patients outside of the hospital with oral antibiotics. Increasing evidence suggests that most patients should be treated with intravenous antibiotics in order to offer the best chance for saving the fallopian tubes.

When a fertilized egg cannot move properly through the tube, it is likely to implant in the wall of the tube and develop as a tubal or ectopic pregnancy. Currently, there is an epidemic of ectopic pregnancies in the United States — 30,000 each year — and chlamydial infection is one of the major causes. Another consequence of PID is chronic pelvic pain which occurs in 20-25% of all women with this infection. Billions of dollars are spent annually to pay for the consequences of chlamydial infection.

Chlamydia infection in pregnancy has been associated with an increased chance of preterm labor which would result in a premature baby such as Brenda's. If a baby is delivered through an infected cervix, the infant's eyes may be infected resulting in a discharge of pus from the eyes. Fortunately, this infection also responds well to antibiotic treatment. This is one of the reasons why newborn babies have antibiotic ointment placed in their eyes after birth.

Brenda's Future

A young woman attempting to live her life as a Christian, Brenda was victimized by the selfish, sinful acts of others. A baby was dead and a young mother devastated.

Brenda was not a quitter. Her infection was successfully treated with tetracycline. She began to put her life back together slowly. She found strength and comfort in her personal relationship with Christ. The church continued to be the focal point of the lives of Brenda and her daughter. The young mother returned to school and graduated from a nurses' training program. She is now a successful registered nurse and is planning to be married to a wonderful Christian businessman.

Reflections and Perspectives

by Donald M. Joy

It doesn't seem fair that Brenda could have been carrying an infection that would kill her baby and destroy her fertility without her noticing something really was wrong with the pregnancy. How could God allow such a tragedy without warning?

There is a Christian principle which links wrong acts to wrong consequences. We know, for example, that rape and sexual violence are always "wrong" even though somebody might say what is happening is "fun." So "wrongness" is based on consequences.

We often use sarcasm, for example, because a clever joke at somebody's expense is really hilarious fun. But the effect on the person and on our future relationship with that person gives us a clear indication that sarcasm is sin. So there are a lot of sexual sins because there are a lot of valuable personal domains that can be damaged or destroyed: feelings of attraction, of affection, of commitment, of inspired faithfulness and so forth. These are all "at risk" when someone runs a Mack truck through the flower garden.

The unfortunate thing about sin of any kind is that we have to wait for the "harvest" to get the bottom line information on what it cost and who had to pay. Brenda felt violated by Sam's forced penetration. She knew immediately that this effort at being sexual as husband and wife was sinful simply because it trampled important values. But human sexuality also contains the domains associated with reproduction: fertility, potential for unlimited possible combinations of new life and personality and the stuff for creating a person to inhabit eternity. The pregnancy that resulted from the forced intercourse invaded the eternity supermarket and selected a unique person for life. That newly created life was a glorious "good" not a "sin," but the conditions surrounding the impregnating event were criminal.

And the chlamydia? That was pure sin. In the most invasive, vulnerable, intimate and "death like" moments of ecstasy, sexually transmitted diseases inhabit the inner sanctuary where eternity and life processes are brought together. So when anyone fools around by having sex with a series of people just for kicks, the "dis-ease" is a symptom that something is dreadfully wrong with the players in this drama. You could say that all STDs are consequences of "diseased" people, relationships and exploitation of other folks. Brenda must have sensed her vulnerability to "becoming unequally joined" to a bad player, so she was refusing to have sex with her demanding husband. But she and the baby bore the consequences of his playing around with the stuff of life. He pays, too, but we have lost track of him and his continuing saga of pain and grief.

How can you call Sam's demand for sex a "rape"? Where do sexual rights fit into a marriage?

Sexual intimacy begins with respect, high communication and the uniting of common vision and dreams for present and future. Sex without those components is either "porn" sex (exploitation of one person by another or of two people scratching each others' backs only for personal gratification) or "rape" (stealing sex against the other person's will). We call "porn" sex an arrangement for mutually consenting adults, and even some marriages never achieve real intimacy and hold together by episodes of mutual self-gratification of the sexual impulses of the partners. We call rape the forcible performance of sexual favors, acts or of passive surrender to be used sexually. Rape occurs on the street or anywhere, including within marriage. Brenda's report is a case of sexual violence within marriage.

Sam's bid for group sex is an early clue that he is a *porneia* man. That Greek word gave us "pornography," but it also gave us the old King James Bible word "fornication." A "pornicator" in that Bible sense is a person who is out for sexual pleasure and sees people as objects to use in any way that satisfies him. The Bible uses a feminine noun which gets translated "harlot" or "prostitute" and builds from the same "porn" base. The masculine noun translates as "whoremonger." Fornication is nowhere limited to premarital sex, but most often refers to adult, married, even managerial or royal men and women who decided to "do it MY way." Rape is a violent form of "porn," which refuses to play the game or pay the participant, demanding sexual performance and often seizing it violently.

But both the "porn" and "rape" versions of sexual activity miss the high ground of respect-based sexual communication. Read the Song of Songs, sometimes called the Song of Solomon, in the Old Testament for a powerful love song with explicit sexual dimensions. Notice that the speeches of the husband and wife to each other build them up by adoring each other, praising the virtues and the excellence of body build and of sexual anatomy. It is in the spirit of such sexual communication and celebration that the Apostle Paul advised the early Christians:

> The husband should give to his wife her conjugal rights, and likewise the wife to her husband. For the wife does not rule over her own body, but the husband does; likewise the husband does not rule over his own body, but the wife does. Do not refuse one another except perhaps by agreement for a season, that you may devote yourselves to prayer; but then come together again, lest Satan tempt you through lack of self-control (1 Corinthians 7:3-5, RSV).

In this chapter we have reflected on the tragic breakdown of Brenda and Sam's relationship. It was flawed by Sam's invisible hungers for sex which broke down the barriers which protect a husband and wife's ultimate vulnerability — being naked and without shame. The unhappy sequence of events which led to the violent end of the marriage and deadly and crippling infection make us cry out, "How much worse could life get?"

Brenda has the courage to play out her remaining options with grace and courage. We celebrate her recovery.

Chapter Five

Beside the Old Gray Barn

by W. David Hager, M.D.

When my wife, Linda, and I were dating, we frequently enjoyed going on picnics in the country. One of our favorite spots was a picturesque stream running beside an old gray barn on a farm in the bluegrass region of central Kentucky. We loved to talk about our relationship and our future while aimlessly throwing pebbles into the brook. The small stones would drop into the water and sink undisturbed, but the ripples they caused seemed to go on endlessly. One pebble could have an effect on water far away from the initial site of contact.

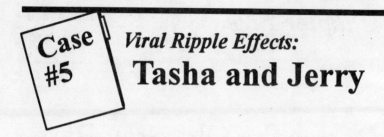

Viral Ripple Effects: Tasha and Jerry

I thought about the ripple effect when I listened to the story of Tasha and Jerry in my office. Jerry is a former substance abuser who experienced a dramatic Christian conversion. He subsequently spent 18 months in a drug rehabilitation program, went back to school, graduated from college and is now working toward a masters degree in social work.

Jerry met my patient, Tasha, while they were in college. They were married soon after graduation, and Tasha began teaching elementary school to help put Jerry through graduate school. Unexpectedly, Tasha became pregnant when she forgot to take her birth control pills with her on a trip, and they did not use backup contraception. They were disappointed at the timing, but agreed that as Christians, abortion certainly was not an option.

Contracting Hepatitis B

Today, we screen all pregnant women for hepatitis B during pregnancy, but, at the time that Tasha was pregnant several years ago, this was not routine practice. During the time when he was abusing drugs, Jerry had been exposed to hepatitis B virus while sharing needles with a friend. Jerry was unaware that he had been infected. Although not obviously ill, he carried the organism in his body.

Although hepatitis B is usually transmitted via in-fected blood, it is possible for the organism to be trans-mitted during sexual intercourse in seminal fluid. Tasha was also unaware that she had been infected by her hus-band. With no admitted risk factors, neither of them had been tested for the virus.

Deadly Effect

Tasha delivered a healthy baby boy. Everything was fine until the child was 18 months old. At that time, his parents noted a marked decrease in his growth rate and distention of his abdomen. They took him to his pediatri-cian who found a large tumor in the baby's liver. Surgery followed in an attempt to remove the mass from the liver, however, the surface of the liver had ruptured. Widespread cancer was found in the child's abdomen. Their son died three months later, in spite of chemo-therapy, from cancer of the liver.

Prognosis for Hepatitis B

Hepatitis B virus is an organism that is usually transmit-ted in a blood-borne manner. It is possible, however, for the virus to be spread through other body fluids. Persons may be infected with hepatitis and develop a rapidly progressive disease that overcomes the individual's de-fenses against infection and results in death from the effects on the liver and other vital organs. Other people may be exposed to the virus and either overcome the infection or become carriers of the virus as Jerry did.

Persons infected with the hepatitis B virus may de-velop tiredness, weakness, loss of appetite and changes in the color of the skin or the mucous membranes of the eyes. Carriers may have no symptoms at all.

When Tasha's baby was later diagnosed with hepatocellular cancer of the liver, both parents were tested for the virus and found to be positive for hepatitis B. Thus Jerry had infected Tasha via intercourse, and Tasha had infected their baby through the exchange of blood across the placenta during pregnancy.

There is no definitive cure for hepatitis. Patients must have supportive treatment when ill and be advised of the possibility of spread of the virus to others. When a mother is found to be infected with the virus on blood tests, it is necessary to give her newborn baby Hepatitis B Immune Globulin, a vaccine to protect the baby from active infection and to prevent the child from becoming a carrier.

Physicians and other health care workers face a tremendous risk from infection with hepatitis B virus. There are 300,000 new cases of hepatitis B in the U. S. annually. As a result of this infection, there are 4,800 deaths in the general population. Some 12,000 to 18,000 health care workers are infected each year as a result of exposure to patients' blood, resulting in 250 deaths. This virus poses a greater threat to physicians in the number infected and the mortality rate from such infection than the HIV virus presently does.

Tasha and Jerry: Prognosis

When Tasha and Jerry were counseled about the cause of their baby's cancer, Jerry became withdrawn and began to abuse drugs again. Shortly thereafter, he began to physically abuse Tasha, and she had to seek police protection. They are now in marriage counseling and Jerry is back in a rehabilitation program. Tasha is teaching to support her family.

Jerry made a bad choice in his youth. The ripples of his behavior affected many other people, including his innocent wife and child and the grandparents who loved their grandchild so much. Although we can receive forgiveness for our past sins, we are not promised that we will not suffer the consequences of our behavior. Fortunately for Jerry and all of us, we *are* promised that we can be delivered from the darkness of our lives (Colossians 1:13-14):

> For he has rescued us from the domain of darkness and transferred us into the kingdom of His beloved Son, in whom we have redemption, the forgiveness of sins (NASB).

We do not have to repeat our behavior of the past.

Reflections and Perspectives

by Donald M. Joy

Why did it take physicians so long to begin testing for hepatitis B? Isn't the loss of Tasha's and Jerry's baby partly the fault of medical authorities?

If you take a minute to contemplate how many new viruses and diseases have appeared in the last 10 years, you get the idea that the human race is running into more and bigger trouble. Hepatitis B was a rare problem, a risk largely limited to health care professionals working around patients and their blood, until the 1960s saw hundreds of thousands of drug users turning to needles on the street.

It is true that Tasha's and Jerry's lost baby was partly a matter of "timing" in medical practice. Indeed, the very idea that physicians "practice" suggests that our physical and medical problems are so complicated, so unique and so changing that no doctor will ever really "get it all down." (I advise my students that ministry is the same way— we are always learning, always practicing the cure of souls.)

Looked at morally and ethically, it is easy to conclude that humans are profoundly complicated. As their choices expand, so also will their risks. For example, as we probe space and contemplate life beyond this planet, one of the greatest medical fears involves what contamination — viruses and diseases — we may import from materials brought back to us from other environments.

It doesn't seem fair that Tasha and Jerry should be trapped by Jerry's past behav-

ior. Why doesn't God cure people of past diseases when they come to faith and a life of godly discipleship?

As a Christian physician, Dr. Hager feels the grief you express. As he opens his casebook for you, he is intentionally exposing issues which trouble both his patients and him very deeply. The first "rule" of medical practice, in this case, lines up with the first "rule" of God's creation. Jerry's wild and crazy past caught up with him. The virus he took into his body eventually spread agony throughout his young family. It now lingers in the wings, ready to walk on stage with any future pregnancy or to show up in either his or Tasha's body when they may become easy victims to a latent virus they carry.

We need to reflect on the fact that we can always reduce the risk of viral or bacterial infection by getting back to basics and by simplifying the behavior. The life of honesty, peace, fidelity and healthy diet always predicts health, resistance to viruses and infections and long life. Christian scriptures express this virtue of simplicity as minding our parents:

> Children, obey your parents in the Lord, for this is right. "Honor your father and mother" — which is the first commandment with a promise — "that it may go well with you and that you may enjoy long life on the earth" (Ephesians 6:1-3).

But in the older Jewish Scriptures — our Old Testament — health and protection from viruses and other diseases is also put under the condition of absolute trust and fidelity to God. The idea is that if we live our lives making all decisions based on God's values, commands and preferences, we will be using our bodies according to the manufacturer's instructions, so we will be free of diseases ususally transmitted sexually. Look at Psalm 91:

He who dwells in the shelter of the Most High
will rest in the shadow of the Almighty.
I will say of the Lord, "He is my refuge and my fortress,
my God, in whom I trust."
Surely he will save you from the fowler's snare
and from the deadly pestilence.
He will cover you with his feathers,
and under his wings you will find refuge;
his faithfulness will be your shield and rampart.
You will not fear the terror of night,
nor the arrow that flies by day,
nor the pestilence that stalks in the darkness,
nor the plague that destroys at midday.
A thousand may fall at your side,
ten thousand at your right hand,
but it will not come near you.
You will only observe with your eyes
and see the punishment of the wicked.
If you make the Most high your dwelling —
even the Lord, who is my refuge —
then no harm will befall you,
no disaster will come near your tent.
For he will command his angels concerning you
to guard you in all your ways;
They will lift you up in their hands
so that you will not strike your foot
against a stone.
You will tread upon the lion and the cobra;
you will trample the great lion and the serpent.
"Because he loves me," says the Lord,

"I will rescue him;
I will protect him, for
he acknowledges my
name.
He will call upon me, and
I will answer him;
I will be with him in
trouble,
I will deliver him and
honor him.
With long life will I satisfy him
and show him my sal-
vation."

Unfortunately, good
people still get struck down
by cancer, and other viruses
and infections, but at a remarkably lower frequency.
So we can rest in the comfort that the principle of simplicity and obedience to the
Creator's Manual works
very well. But we are also
grateful that medical science
becomes increasingly careful and skeptical and runs
tests routinely to provide
early detection, to save life,
and to prolong it in the face
of terrifying diseases.

In this chapter Jerry's virus transmitted to Tasha and
to their lost baby provides a
stark reminder that we do
live in a booby-trapped
world where thieves and
robbers and viruses can
creep in and blow our lives
apart. We have reflected on
the importance of life-long
sensitivity to how fragile and
precious life is and how
connected we are at all
times to the future members
of the human family. As an
ethicist and a theologian
outside the medical profession, I urge you to give
thanks for the accelerating
net of protective testing that
physicians are casting about
us in an age when viruses
and infections are prolifer-
ating at a staggering rate.

Chapter Six

Recognizing the Dark Side

by W. David Hager, M.D.

As a young physician, I frequently saw patients who were suffering from the consequences of their behavior as a result of destructive choices. Although I diagnosed and treated these people appropriately, I experienced great difficulty in being loving and forgiving when it seemed to me that they were only reaping the consequences they deserved.

With time, God has worked in my life as I have moved with him into an intense journey of spiritual and emotional wholeness. A part of that journey has included acknowledging my own dark side, a side that had been filled with pride and egotism. This journey has also included the realization that my capacity for sin is as great as anyone else's. In recognizing this, I have been able to become more forgiving of others. As Dr. David Seamands has said, forgiveness is ". . .the key relational issue of the Bible."

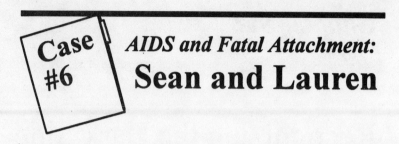

AIDS and Fatal Attachment:
Sean and Lauren

I saw true love and forgiveness exemplified by Lauren, a 27-year-old wife of a graduate student. Lauren met Sean when they were attending college and they were married during her junior year. Early in their relationship, she had been concerned about Sean's limited interest in her sexually, but blamed the pressures of school and the stress of trying to get into graduate school. Her fears were enhanced when they only had intercourse once on their honeymoon and seldom thereafter.

Two years into their marriage, during one of their infrequent times of sexual intercourse, Lauren conceived. Sean became extremely withdrawn. Finally, Lauren confronted him with her fears about his sexual behavior and appetite. Sean admitted that he was bisexual and had been involved across the years — before marriage and since — in several homosexual relationships.

Lauren was appalled, but instead of lashing out at Sean with bitterness and anger, she responded with love and forgiveness. She encouraged her husband to seek counseling for sexual addiction and to become involved with a small group of students and professors in a program focusing on emotional and spiritual wholeness.

Ask the Doctor

At the time of her first prenatal obstetric visit, Lauren hesitantly revealed this information to me and requested a blood test for AIDS (Acquired Immune Deficiency Syndrome). Her blood test returned from the laboratory with a positive result. Confirmatory tests were also positive. Subsequently, Sean was also tested. Both his screening and confirmatory tests were also positive. This meant that their unborn child would have a significant chance (13-39%) of being infected with HIV (Human Immunodeficiency Virus) and at high risk for developing AIDS.

In spite of the horrifying impact of these results, Lauren continued to show love and respect for Sean and demonstrated a profound spirit of forgiveness toward him. Her love and commitment were unlike any I had ever seen. She attributed it not to herself, but to her willingness to allow God to love through her.

AIDS Today

AIDS was originally thought to be a disease of active homosexual or "gay" males. Now we realize that heterosexual transmission is possible by transfer of infected body fluids such as semen. It is estimated that more than 10 percent of all AIDS cases are heterosexually transmitted. Sexual transmission and intravenous drug abuse (which transfers the virus by contaminated needles or blood) are the two principal ways by which women are infected, although they may also, in rare cases, be infected from an infected blood transfusion.

As of June, 1992, more than 500,000 cases of AIDS were reported to the World Health Organization, with

230,179 of those coming from the United States. Approximately 1.5 of every 1,000 pregnant women in the U.S. are HIV positive. In the U.S., 1,954 cases have been reported in children under 13 years of age. Although the mortality rate is published as 67%, there are no long-term survivors.

We are still learning a great deal about AIDS and the virus which causes it. If a person is exposed to Human Immunodeficiency Virus (HIV) and infected by this virus, most will have developed a positive HIV test within 12 months, the majority in the first six months. On the other hand, of those with a positive HIV test, it may take seven to ten years or more for 50% of them to develop the disease called AIDS. During the incubation period for the disease — the time from exposure to the virus until AIDS develops — there may be no symptoms of the virus. The first warning may come only when the patient develops a severe infection which overwhelms the immune system leaving the disease to run its course.

Can women rely on their spouse or sexual partner to tell them if they are HIV positive? In two studies, 52% and 97% respectively indicated they would not inform their partners and would proceed with sexual activity.

Infection with HIV causes a reversal of the normal ratio of good and bad lymphocytes, a white blood cell in the blood stream that helps to combat infection. Patients are unable to fight infections and cancer. "Cause of death" may officially be listed as one of these other diseases, such as *Pneumocyostis carinii* pneumonia, toxoplasmosis or Kaposi's sarcoma.

A great deal of time and money is being spent to

develop a treatment for AIDS. At present, a drug called Azothymidine (AZT) is being used to attempt to slow the progression of the disease. It may also be used to "prophylax" persons who are HIV positive but have not developed AIIDS. The search for a cure for AIDS continues, but like other viruses, there is no antibiotic that will cure the disease. There is also work being done to develop an effective vaccine. We presently treat and contain other viruses, many of which are not life threatening, but we do not have a "cure" for any sexually transmitted virus at this time.

Pregnancy and AIDS Transmission

Women who are pregnant and have a positive HIV test have a 13-39% chance of transmitting the disease to their newborn baby. The more advanced the disease is at the time of pregnancy, the greater the chance of transmission to the baby. The more severely ill the mother is during pregnancy, the greater the chance of transmission to the baby. The mortality rate among infants and children with AIDS is extremely high. Unfortunately, avoiding a vaginal delivery and doing a cesarean section does not alter the transmission from mother to baby at all. Eighty-five percent of women who are found to have AIDS while pregnant elect to continue their pregnancies.

Baby with HIV?

Lauren delivered a healthy baby boy nine months after her diagnosis. The baby's blood test was HIV positive because of the transfer of blood from mother to baby.

The infant was followed for six months and the tests continued to remain positive. In non-infected babies, the test will eventually become negative.

Lauren showed remarkable constraint as she faced the knowledge about her husband's addiction, and the fact that he had infected her and their baby with HIV. The baby is showing some early evidence that he may be developing AIDS, and yet she loves and forgives her husband completely. Lauren has given me an opportunity to reflect on what it means to love unconditionally as Jesus demanded.

Reflections and Perspectives

by Donald M. Joy

Some of the toughest decisions I have monitored involved issues of betrayal, marital and sexual fraud, and questions of forgiveness. When a person is a victim of deception, and especially when the deception is accompanied by invasive disease introduced under the guise of intimacy, rage is an appropriate response.

Is a person supposed to forgive and forget if a spouse is promiscuous and keeps coming back and wanting to "start over"? Give me a break! Is Lauren required by God or Jesus to forgive Sean and his homosexual promiscuity and take him back? I suppose you will quote Jesus and tell her to forgive him "even to seventy times seven times"!

God loves unconditionally and Jesus uses God's unconditional and perfect love for everybody as a model for how we are to love.

"You have heard that it was said, 'Love your neighbor and hate your enemy.' But I tell you: Love your enemies and pray for those who persecute you, that you may be sons of your Father in heaven. He causes his sun to rise on the evil and the good, and sends rain on the righteous and the unrighteous. If you love those who love you, what reward will you get? Are not even the tax collectors doing that? And if you greet only your brothers, what are you doing more than others? Do not even pagans do that? Be perfect, therefore, as your heavenly Father is perfect" (Matthew 5:43-48).

But God doesn't "become one flesh" with anybody. It is this one flesh contact which can defraud and turn out to be fornication. And fornication, Jesus says, breaks the one flesh bond so profoundly that there is no risk of committing adultery if the victim remarries:

". . . anyone who divorces his wife, except for marital unfaithfulness, causes her to commit adultery, and anyone who marries a woman so divorced commits adultery" (Matthew 5:32).

"Fornication" is the "porn" word I mentioned in an earlier chapter, and Sean is a classic fornicator. He goes for the thrill with a series of homosexual partners while at the same time being sexual with Lauren to whom he is married. Dr. Hager rightly referred him to therapy for sexual addiction.

Lauren chose to practice unconditional love with Sean. Nobody said it was an easy choice. Lauren had been defrauded, sexually used within her marriage and infected with the fatal HIV/AIDS virus before she learned of Sean's homosexual behavior.

Lauren and Sean now have a child and are hoping that somehow the baby will turn up HIV negative in a few months. In the worst case scenario, there are three premature fatal illnesses in their family's future. Lauren's options now are to abandon the marriage and leave with the child as a protest against Sean's fatal fraud, or go down in flames together in a voluntary self-sacrifice as if she had willingly infected herself because of her love for him.

There is no reason, however, for anyone to risk HIV/AIDS or any disease or loss of integrity for sexual love. Indeed, the honest human would refuse to become sexual without marriage and full disclosure of both sexual histories, backed up by the best medical perspective and prognosis. "I love you too much to get sexual with you until we know everything about each other and until we can verify that we are clean for each other" is the urgently needed "proposal" today.

I listened to a young woman's reasoning and was dumbfounded: "If I am ever going to get HIV, I've probably already got it, so I don't want to know." That kind of warped reasoning is rampant among the compulsively addicted.

Remember that in Chapter Two I caution folks to go slow on forgiveness. You cannot quickly forgive as though forgiveness were a button you could push on an elevator. Count the cost first. Be sure you understand your losses and see the future probable costs.

"Cheap forgiveness" is only words, masks the loss in denial and actually postpones the healing and forgiveness that can be offered only when the grieving is completed.

Costly forgiveness eventually commutes the sentence which should rightly fall on the guilty. To forgive is to say, "I paid twice. The first time was when you lied, deceived and defrauded me. Now I'm going to take the blame and the penalty on myself; it is as if I did it to myself. I forgive you." Any other kind of forgiveness will not last and is only another form of denial, no matter how cleverly we disguise our rage, resentment and pride.

Jesus paid twice for our sins. He paid once when we stiffened our necks and determined to "do it our way." But Jesus paid again when he said, "Lay all of

their sin to my account."
That is why it cost the Son
of God his life! In Jesus'
case, we got to go free. In
Lauren's case they will
likely recover their peace together as they forgive themselves and each other.
Forgiveness is a choice, not
an automatic response be-
cause someone is religious.

*How did we get in this
AIDS mess? Were the doc-
tors asleep at the switch?*

Doctors and medical re-
search people are always being confronted by new and
stronger diseases and strains
of viruses. You are on to
something when you as-
sume that AIDS is a new
problem. The more experi-
ence we have with disease,
the better our medical science. So we are always op-
timistic that we will make a
breakthrough that will cure
or at least control the new
diseases and new strains.

However, I regret to re-
mind you, as Dr. Hager said,
we still have no cure for any
virus. Your childhood
chickenpox, for example,
was a virus called varicella,
and it remains in your body.
If your immune system
weakens — perhaps be-
cause of an illness or unusual stress — it often
reappears with a chickenpox
rash of blistered sores. This
reappearance of the old virus is usually called shingles.

We know that human life
and health is remarkably
precious, normally resistant
to disease, but always fragile. So it becomes a unique
human moral responsibility
to practice healthy living
patterns. The connection between health, wholeness
and holiness is very close.
But the connection between
disease, devastation and ir-
responsibility is also very
close. Innocent victims get
caught in the cross-fire.
With many diseases it is easy
to draw a line back to their
origin and see that they

flourished because people were careless, unsanitary or stepped across boundaries of constructive human behavior.

Since humans tend to be careless and to break the boundaries of what is healthful, we can expect that viruses will continue to rise and breed new strains. Doctors cannot anticipate what new threat is around the corner.

This whole AIDS disaster really bothers me. Part of the time I'm angry at the drug addicts and active homosexuals because of all of the innocent people they infect when they decide to spread their fatal HIV disease by sexual contact or to make a little money selling their blood!

It is appropriate for you to be angry. All of us are at risk when a few people break the health boundaries and set off an epidemic. In the case of AIDS, they are unleashing a fatal plague. Anger, by itself, doesn't change a sex addict's behavior, but it can lead to social, political and scientific revolution focused on bringing responsibility back into the human community.

I spoke of boundaries in response to the first question. It is clear that exclusive monogamy established between healthy virgins is the Creation way to elminiate all sexually transmitted viruses and diseases. There were early speculations about where the HIV came from. We do know that it is carried in some animal species without turning into AIDS. We know that the drug communities spread it with contaminated needles as they mixed blood. We know that some homosexual practices spread HIV. But the promiscuity, incest and rape statistics in our culture are the unrelenting red flags of warning we must watch. HIV is now spreading downward to our teen population, and unless we undergo a major cultural change in sexual behavior, we will find HIV and AIDS invading all of our communities and families.

Look at "boundaries." Food preparation rules or laws are put in place to make good health predictable. Any tribe which fails to generate healthful laws of food preparation is planting the seeds of disease and death.

In an even more obvious way, unless sexual behavior is personally harnessed and restricted to exclusive marriage boundaries, it will be gathering diseases and spreading them. Sexually transmitted diseases tend to attack and destroy fertility — a sort of reciprocal reward in which the destructive behavior is paid back by destroying the organs at the heart of the issue. That rule is written everywhere in the universe. The Bible observes — but does not flaunt or harrass anyone — that the person who sins dies. "The wages of sin is death" (Romans 6:23). So we are not surprised that careful observers, like E. Stanley Jones, are always reminding us that anything that "goes against life" is sin and anything that is sin "goes against life." "E-V- I-L," Jones loves to say, "is L-I-V-E" turned around backwards.

As a boy I learned Edwin Markham's famous poem.

> The robber is robbed by
> his riches.
> The tyrant is dragged by
> his chain.
> The schemer is snared by
> his cunning.
> The slayer lies dead by
> the slain.

So your anger is a good first step. But you will find

no pleasure in the death of victims of AIDS or crack cocaine, or any other form of E-V-I-L, even though the confused, desperate and addicted people may have originally made choices which set them on the road toward their fatal addiction.

In this painful chapter, Dr. Hager has opened the door on a very complicated HIV/AIDS case. We have faced the fact that going against the rules always leads to suffering and loss, but rarely so surely or so quickly as with exposure to the HIV package of trouble. Here, as always, it is easy to appeal for lifelong integrity, honesty and exclusive sexual commitment.

Chapter Seven

Silence in the Pool

by W. David Hager, M.D.

In 1976 Linda and I had been married for six years, and
our oldest son, Philip, was three years old. We decided
to vacation in Florida that summer and visit with my
closest friend, Steve Davis. Philip loved Steve and
followed him everywhere he went.

We had a delightful, refreshing vacation. One hot
summer evening, Steve and I decided to go out to the
pool and cool off. Naturally, Philip wanted to be included in this activity with the men. We laced Philip up
in his life jacket and dived into the cool water for a
swim. Ever the adventurer, Philip howled in delight as
we tossed him around in the water. Quickly an hour had
passed, and it was time to return to the house.

Philip climbed up the steps and onto the pool deck.
Steve and I stayed in the shallow end of the pool talking
about football games and girlfriends of the past. Soon
we turned to get out of the water and called for Philip,
but there was no answer, only a deafening silence.
Suddenly, Steve cried out, "He's on the bottom!" He
plunged to the bottom of the pool, grabbed Philip and

threw him to me on the deck.

Before I could stop to think, I instinctively began CPR on my only son. In and out I breathed. I firmly compressed his tiny chest. He did not move. After what seemed a lifetime, but actually was only seconds, he began to squirm and breathe. Anxiously, I watched as life awakened in his motionless body.

While we had been talking, Philip evidently had taken off his life jacket and slipped back into the water. Apparently, he lost his balance on the steps and went under. Steve and I were completely unaware of the potential consequences of our inattention.

I was reminded of this frightening event when I heard about the consequences of group B streptococcal infection in the lives of Dave and Jamie.

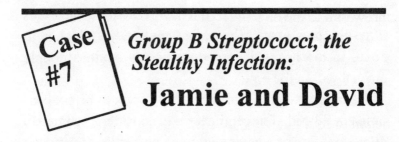

Case #7

Group B Streptococci, the Stealthy Infection:

Jamie and David

Jamie and Dave were married shortly after they completed their senior year in college. They had dated since they were sophomores. Their enthusiasm and vigor for life was contagious and they were very popular.

Dave was hired by the local branch of a large national electronics corporation. Jamie began to teach elementary school in a nearby school district. They worked hard, enjoyed their life together and made plans for their future.

After three years of marriage, Jamie became pregnant. The young couple was ecstatic at the thought of having their first child. Jamie stayed physically fit and busied herself with decorating the nursery. Dave was an excellent cabinet maker and started building a new cherry crib.

Premature Delivery

The pregnancy was uncomplicated until the thirty-second week of pregnancy. Forty-weeks is normally full term. Jamie began having a strange tightening around her back and lower abdomen. Because she was only 32 weeks pregnant, she reasoned that the tightening must be Braxton-Hicks contractions — pre-term contractions which do not cause the cervix to dilate — and not true labor.

After eight hours, the frequency of the tightening was three minutes apart. She called me, and I told her to come to the hospital immediately. The anxious couple arrived within the hour.

I examined Jamie and found her cervix to be six centimeters dilated. Ten centimeters is considered complete dilatation. She was having uterine contractions every two minutes. At six centimeters, she was too far dilated to attempt to stop her labor. Within two hours she was completely dilated and ready to deliver.

The neonatologist was called, and Jamie was prepared for delivery. Within minutes, I held a three-pound, five ounce baby boy in my hands as I clamped and cut the umbilical cord and rushed him to the waiting neonatology team for resuscitation. Babies delivered at this early gestation frequently are not capable of breathing on their own and must be placed on a ventilator. Jamie and Dave's son had the resuscitation tube placed into the trachea to allow a hand-held oxygen bag or a machine to breathe for him, and the neonatologist began administering intravenous fluids. The baby was critically ill.

Group B Streptococci

Unknown to her, Jamie carried a bacteria called group B streptococci in her vagina. Thirty percent of all pregnant women carry this organism. It may exist in the vagina quiescently or it may move into the amnionic membranes that surround the amnionic fluid and the baby. If the strep infection takes this more active pattern, it may appear as disease in the mother or be transmitted to the newborn child at the time of delivery. In some cases the infection actively attacks both mother and child. Fortunately the attack rate of infection in babies is only one per 1,000 births. Although it is not considered one of the classic venereal diseases, group B streptococci may be sexually transmitted and frequently mother and father are both infected. The organism has been associated with preterm labor and premature rupture of the membranes in pregnancy.

When babies are infected with group B streptococci before or at delivery, they may develop pneumonia, meningitis or infection in the blood stream called bacteremia. Although the organism is sensitive to treatment with penicillin antibiotics, sometimes the infection is so far advanced that the infant's infection cannot be cured. Severe infection with this organism carries a high mortality rate.

Survival Scramble

The tiny baby that I handed to the neonatologist was infected with this bacterial species. Jamie and Dave were panic stricken. At first they denied that this could be happening to their child. Soon they began to search for cures, just as I frantically had started CPR on Philip. They sought second opinions and insisted on transfer of the baby to another institution, which was carried out rapidly. Even these events did nothing to alter the course of the fatal process. In spite of all of our technology with ventilators, intravenous fluids, antibiotics and vascular support medications, the baby's strep could not be cured, and he died 30 hours after he was delivered.

Jamie and Dave were completely unaware that they carried this organism. We had no reason to suspect that she was a high risk patient.

Since Jamie has had one child infected with group B streptococci she may be colonized with the bacteria. In a subsequent pregnancy, that child could possibly be infected. We will screen her with cultures during her next pregnancy. If they are positive, she will receive ampicillin just before and at delivery to decrease the chance of transmission of the infection to the baby.

Recovery from Devastation

The unexpected loss of their firstborn devastated the young couple. With counseling and prayer, they are recovering from their grief. They plan to have another child, but I am encouraging them to bring closure to this sad chapter in their lives and not attempt to replace a loss with another baby too quickly.

Steve and I had no idea when we went swimming that night in Florida what would happen to Philip. Although we knew that unattended children could drown in a pool, we were totally unaware that we were being inattentive to Philip. Even when our intentions are ideal, we may face unfavorable consequences.

Reflections and Perspectives

by Donald M. Joy

What kind of a world is it when you can be carrying a disease over which you have no control and show no symptoms that can take the life of your innocent child?

Jamie's and Dave's loss of their baby raises this question, which all of us who are thoughtful have to ask.

We have grown up in an affluent culture where babies tend to live and thrive and the boundaries of lifespan are being pushed further and further until birthday greetings are broadcast daily to many folks well beyond a hundred years of age. We have come to believe that all diseases have a cure, that we are invincible.

But the fact is, we live in a world that is bent and deformed. Death and decay are mixed with the grounding of new life. Without well-developed health sciences and ecological watchdogging of the world's central tendency toward death, perhaps half of newborns would die before reaching two years of age, and the lifespan for the survivors would be 50 years or less.

These pessimistic facts help you and me to adjust our eyes and our judgment. We all need to adopt a habit of living defensively against what we have come to call natural disaster. Besides living in a hostile environment with uncertain and often violent weather, we walk and breathe daily in a literal battlefield of hostile microscopic organisms, and viruses which threaten to bring us down to death and decay. That's why we teach our youngsters basic rules of sanitation before they can talk. We vote for their survival. And while we take specific aim on life-threatening diseases and invest enormous energy and money in trying to eradicate them, there is always the odd chance that our best efforts will not find a cure. Even when we hold a disease at bay, a stray bullet of an infection or a virus will slip past our best protection and take us or our baby away.

So, congratulations for asking one of those real and tough questions. You've seen the dark side of our broken world. We'll all be walking softly, avoiding unnecessary risks, praying for breakthroughs and the courage to live by the knowledge we already have, and trying to survive when we lose a baby, a child, a teen, a spouse or anyone at all.

In the Creation account, God did not create evil or death. Evil and death are always aliens to God's purposes, always intruders. We have every reason to resist them. Theologians wrestle with the "why?" and "how?" questions and call the work "theodicy." They often speak of "Fall" and even "curse" as the origin of evil. When theodicy goes to Broadway, Eugene O'Neill said it simply, but powerfully, in *The Great God Brown*, when he observed that "humans are born broken; they spend their lives mending. The grace of God is the glue."

Frankly, I'm not sure I would want to risk another pregnancy if I had lost a baby to this stealth killer in my body. I admire Jamie's and Dave's courage. Where does it come from?

Let me respond in two

layers. First, the fact is that we live in a contaminated universe — a broken world, as I mentioned in response to the first question. We are aware of that, generally. We remember not to drink water unless we are sure it has been purified. We want to buy fresh vegetables from sources we can trust to have protected them during growth and handling so as to keep them free from infections or chemicals. Meanwhile, within our bodies lurk organisms which are knocking at the door of our systems to reduce us to death. As we stay basically healthy, our immune system does battle with these threatening infections and viruses, mostly winning. It is a little scary to think of this high risk game we play called life.

Second, however, consider this: If we can accept the risks we cope with minute-by-minute to live in this contaminated universe, then we can accept that there are losses worth risking. If we became obsessed with self-protection issues in the face of all of the potential booby traps that could destroy us, we would curl up and die in a corner of some cell or laboratory. Trying to protect ourselves, we would refuse to bring children into the world because it is so full of risk.

But since we have a sense of destiny, of moving toward a better and never-ending existence beyond this earth and life, we are eager to do warfare and battle the forces of evil destruction in this world. We call our children and our acquaintances to join us in this journey of hope. We see life as good, health as worth pursuing and losses worth taking when we are victimized by the crazy evils of this planet.

So Jamie and Dave are grieving now, but looking

for every way to outwit the destructive disease called group B streptococcus and to win the next several rounds because they and their physician have armed themselves. They are smarter now, believing they are resourceful enough to reduce the risks for future pregnancies.

Dr. Hager has wisely urged Dave and Jamie to do their grieving before looking to a second pregnancy. Any loss deserves adequate time invested in reflecting on the reality of the loss, sensing the sorrow, the lost potential, the child who was denied life and the relationship that was cut short by death. This intentional embrace of reality instead of denial by replacement will enrich all of life for them. The lost baby will have provided Jamie and Dave with a curriculum of wisdom that comes only with suffering. They will give themselves permission to be angry at the infection that took their baby. Anger is an essential section of the highway of good grieving. They will need time to sort out what they are angry about.

If they do not take this sorting out time, they are likely to turn to emotional violence on each other, other people or even to abuse a future child. They still need to travel the bargaining, depression and acceptance segments of the grief path. There will be lifelong flashbacks as they briefly revisit that tragic loss of their first baby.

In this chapter, we have faced the frustration and grief of sudden loss by the stealth of group B strep. We have walked with Jamie and Dave through their shock and first response to grief. And we cheer from the stands as they battle an infection we want annihilated from the arsenal of evil.

Chapter Eight

A Stolen Briefcase

by W. David Hager, M.D.

One evening in the early fall, our three sons all had plans to spend the night with separate friends. Linda and I decided to travel to a nearby resort and spend the night just to get away. We had a delightful time together, enjoying each other's company.

The following morning I went out to run, and as I re-entered the parking lot of the hotel I passed our van. Something didn't look right, so I went over and, much to my chagrin, found that someone had broken into our van. A window was shattered. My briefcase with all of my data from a research project was gone. I was planning to write an article based on that research. Apparently the security alarm system had frightened the thieves off, since only my briefcase was taken.

I knew I could reassemble the data from my computer and still write my research, but every time I sat down to work on that project or to write the report I had a deep feeling of anger about being invaded by someone else. I was grateful that nothing else had been stolen. I had the window of the van replaced, but still felt violated by the loss of my prized personal papers and my briefcase. Melanie's story reminded me of those feelings of being violated.

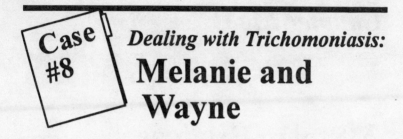

Case #8

Dealing with Trichomoniasis:
Melanie and Wayne

Following my residency in obstetrics and gynecology, I spent two years doing research at the Centers for Disease Control in Atlanta. One of the diseases that I studied was an infection known as trichomoniasis or "trich" (commonly pronounced "trick" in lay terms). Dr . Stuart Brown and I evaluated a single-dose treatment to see if it could adequately replace five- or seven-day treatment regimens.

We saw many patients, male and female, with trich. Our study divided the infected patients into two categories for treatment. One group received the standard seven days of metronidazole (Flagyl) in a dose of 250 mg. three times a day. The other group received a single dose of two grams of the same antibiotic. There was no significant difference in the ability of either regimen to cure the patients with trich. The single dose was adopted as the treatment of choice in the United States.

After starting into the practice of obstetrics and gynecology in 1978, I began to see occasional cases that did not respond to either the single dose or the multiple dose regimens. Even 14- and 21-day regimens failed. Soon other investigators around the country began reporting trichomonas infections that were resistant to metronidazole. My interest in this organism led to the referral of several patients with resistant infections.

Melanie was a 29-year-old teacher when she was referred to my practice. She had grown up in a small town with her parents and two sisters. Melanie was an honor student in high school and received an academic scholarship to college. She graduated from an excellent university as an elementary education major and soon found a job in a new elementary school.

Melanie met Wayne at a party given by one of her friends. They had a great deal in common and soon were seeing each other exclusively. They fell in love and were married one year later. He was handsome and energetic, working hard as a bank vice-president. She was popular with her students and her peers at the school.

A Terrifying Rape

Wayne was out of town frequently on business for the bank. One evening before eating a TV-dinner at home alone, Melanie went for her usual mile and a half run. On a darkened portion of the street where she always ran, Melanie was suddenly grasped by the wrist by a man who reached out from a hiding place behind a clump of bushes. He threw her to the ground, brandished a knife and proceeded to gag and rape her.

Terrified, Melanie struggled to her feet, and staggered home, sobbing quietly. Melanie became frantic and called Wayne. He immediately left his meeting and drove home. He found her disheveled and trembling in their bedroom. Wayne insisted that she go to the local hospital for an evaluation, but Melanie refused, saying, "I am not injured physically, and I don't want people to know." In spite of Wayne's pleadings, she would not comply.

Ten days later, Melanie went to her local gynecologist because she had an abnormal vaginal discharge and vaginal itching. She had not told Wayne about these symptoms. She was diagnosed as having trichomoniasis and was treated with a single oral dose of metroniduzole.

Five days later, her symptoms were unchanged, and she returned to her gynecologist. The same diagnosis was made, and she was treated with a seven-day course of metroniduzole. Still her discharge and itching persisted.

After a third visit, she was referred to my office. Microscopic preparations of the vaginal discharge revealed two distinct types of rounded protozoan organisms with flagella (tails). Melanie had a strain of *Trichomonas vaginalis* which was resistant to standard metroniduzole therapy. I then prescribed an extended course of oral, high dose metroniduzole combined with vaginally administered metroniduzole suppositories, but still Melanie harbored the organisms.

As a last resort, the young school teacher was hospitalized and was treated with intravenous metroniduzole for seven days. Finally, we were able to eradicate the organism, and she was cured. I told Melanie that she must tell Wayne that she had a sexually transmitted disease so that he could be treated. Wayne was horrified but was very understanding and supportive of Melanie. He was treated with high-dose oral metroniduzole at home and was cured as well.

Melanie has received counseling and assistance from the rape crisis center and is in continued therapy. Her determination and her strong faith in a loving and sustaining heavenly Father are enabling her to survive this crisis.

Characteristics of Trich

Trichomoniasis is a vaginal infection caused by *trichomonas vaginalis*, a motile protozoan organism. It is estimated that there are three and one-half to four million new cases in the United States annually. The organism is sexually transmitted by having direct contact with an infected sexual partner. Occasional cases of possible transmission via an infected water supply have been reported.

Once the protozoan gains access to the urethra or vagina in women or the urethra in men, it infects the cells lining those structures. In 70% of cases in women there will be abnormal vaginal discharge, usually thin and foamy or yellowish. In 85% of cases with women there will be vaginal itching. Many men have no symptoms at all, but if they do, they may have symptoms similar to a bladder infection with a burning sensation during urination.

Types of Vaginitis

There are three principal types of vaginitis in women: yeast infections caused by fungi, bacterial vaginosis caused by bacteria that live in the absence of oxygen (*Gardnerella vaginalis, mobilluncus* species and other anaerobic bacteria — bacteria which can live without oxygen), and trichomoniasis. Each of these infections can cause similar symptoms of discharge, burning and itching.

Accurate diagnosis of the type of vaginitis can only be made by taking vaginal specimens (wet-preps) and looking at them under the microscope to identify the causative organisms or by doing specific cultures. Diagnosing the infection based only on symptoms frequently results in errors of diagnosis and poor response to therapy.

Treating Trich

The treatment of choice for trichomonas infections is still metronidazole (Flagyl), an antibiotic which is only effective against anaerobic bacteria. The current regimen of choice is a single, two-gram dose of metronidazole. Patients should be seen back in the office or clinic three to five days after completing therapy for a follow-up wet-prep called a "test of cure." Sexual partners must also be treated since this disease is sexually transmitted.

Some strains of *trichomonas vaginalis,* like Melanie's, now are resistant to normal doses of metronidazole. These resistant strains must be treated with high-dose, extended duration regimens. Currently, we use a combination of vaginal suppositories and high-dose oral therapy. Occasionally it is necessary to use intravenous therapy. Even then, occasional patients cannot be cured and continue to harbor the organism.

Women who are raped should immediately contact a medical care facility equipped for examination of sexually assaulted patients. If the exam is delayed, the information gathered may not be reliable. The exam is done to evaluate for physical trauma, to check for the presence of seminal fluid or sperm and to test for possible sexually transmitted infections. Immediate and follow-up counseling can be arranged with trained counselors and police information can be obtained. Everything possible should be done to assist women in their recovery from this trauma. This is a travesty inflicted on women, and we must reach out to every victim with love and kindness.

Reflections and Perspectives

by Donald M. Joy

Why are women so often the victims of sexual attack? Can't we do anything more to protect them?

Here are some reasons why women are attacked, in a sort of speculative response:

1. Women may be more at peace with their sexuality than men are. Men who attack women sexually are not lovers but angry people. A rape is an episode of power and control by a man who is not at peace with himself and does not see his sexuality as a potential for intimacy and loving.

2. Men are bigger boned, larger and laced with nearly twenty per cent more muscle (by weight!) than women.

3. Women tend to be globally sexual in the sense that they are sexual all over and sexual all of the time; but men tend to be occasionally driven by a sexual appetite and to feel sexual only in the genitals.

The sexes are profoundly different. I've offered three ways that may be related to the tendency for men to be the criminals in sexual assault cases. None of the physiological or psychological differences justifies in any way the pattern of male violence against women. But you asked "why," so I wanted to open the window on some basic possibilities.

The response we must all try to act on, however, is this: Since women are more vulnerable to sexual attack, it becomes urgent for us to assume there is a risk to women who travel alone, run alone, work late at night alone or live alone. Because we live in a broken universe, we simply must "drive" defensively. While we are at the wheel, we must not allow the tragedy of rape to happen easily. Family rape and date rape are particularly troublesome to monitor. So we must teach our daughters to live defensively and assertively because they live among potential rapists.

Young daughters must know that (1) their bodies are their own, and that no one under any circumstance is to touch or force them to touch the parts of the body that are hidden away under a swim suit, (2) they must try to fight off anyone who tries to break that rule and (3) they must report to a parent, or to another trusted authority, anyone who breaks the rule.

Carol Gilligan of Harvard University's moral development center reports another complicating problem. Girls at about age 12 "abandon themselves." They get the message everywhere that *girls must let boys win, excel and have their way* if the girl is to be valued and to find a place in the mixed world of boys and girls. Ironically, the primary "coaches" of this abandoning are women teachers of sixth grade. These teachers encourage boys to be aggressive, to compete and to think critically, but criticize girls as "bossy" or aggressive if they behave in the same self-positive ways.

There is no conspiracy of sixth grade teachers, but there is a universal human problem. Genesis 3:16 cautions the first woman that the man "will rule over" her. But in the story the male dominance comes after the Fall and sin. Whenever a man "rules over a woman," it is always e-v-i-l. It is not God's design, but human default.

The same story tells how the woman's "desire shall be to her husband." If men tend to muscle down women, then women tend to adore, idolize and live their lives for men. The Genesis story contains no simple rape prevention formula, but the woman as victim image can teach us a lot. It can teach us that women, as a group, are likely to abandon themselves, and men are likely to spontaneously put women down. Nothing can be more important for men and women than for them to be aware of this broken aspect of male-female relationships. They should search for marriage partners who will devote a lifetime to correcting the flaw present in both men and women. All other settings, then, need to be kept in focus as potentially dangerous and exploitive, as opening the door to rape.

Together we will continue to rush victims to immediate and continuing medical and therapeutic care, and to rush criminals to exposure and prosecution to the full extent of the law grounded in justice.

I'm baffled why women are so vulnerable to so many sexually transmitted diseases, compared to men who often carry and transmit the diseases but don't know they have them. Is it the "fairness" thing again?

I suggested in the last response that women are "globally sexual." Earlier I referred to the "open system" of female sexuality. I am impressed with the fact that women are the conduit through which all of us make it to this planet alive: through the female sex system. Women are the formation matrix — the Mother — of us all. All of this is another way of observing that a woman's sexuality is her whole personhood. She takes the sperm and ovum and hides them away for nine months and forms the new person inside of herself. This miraculous life cavern simply has to be complicated, sensitive to every invasive intruder, from the host of sperm from which one will be kept in the life business while the others die to the bacteria, viruses and other alien organisms.

In this chapter, Jamie's rape and the resulting stubborn case of "trich" raise the issue of women's vulnerability. Women are vulnerable to rape by men, and they seem to be the victims in disproportionate numbers of the symptoms and consequences of sexually transmitted diseases. I've raised the issue too, in reflection, about how to parent girls to prepare them to be appropriately assertive in dealing with boys and men. We must help them develop habits and social patterns that avoid the solitude that may make them the target of a crazy and probably sexually-diseased male predator.

Chapter Nine

Walking through the Fire

by W. David Hager, M.D.

For the past few years, I have been on a spiritual journey with God. This life-changing experience started several years ago and has intensified as I have been willing to be obedient to his direction in my life. I have had to walk through the fire to get to the healing awaiting me on the other side. A part of this process has involved looking back at events that shaped my childhood, confronting events of the past and bringing them before God in honest confession and repentance.

In January of 1990, I found myself alone in a hotel room in Washington, D.C. the evening before a meeting scheduled to begin the following morning. Recent events had left me agonizing over what the future would hold for me in my marriage, my family, my profession.

I distinctly remember crying out for God's help and sensing his immediate response: "David, I can go no further with you until you are willing to confess, deny yourself and your desire to control everything and obey me."

That was the beginning of the most life-changing

year of my life, and it continues to get better. This could not have occurred had I not been willing to lay down my perceptions of what was important and accept God's design for my life. Confession and repentance were essential to the transformation that has occurred in my life.

I was reminded of this when I reflected on Tina's case.

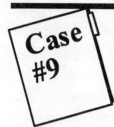

Case #9

Post-Abortion Syndrome and Recovery:
Tina's Story

I recently shared these personal experiences with a young woman named Tina. Tina is 20 years old and very bright, carrying a GPA of 3.45 in college. Tina had not dated often in high school or in her first two years of college. Then she met her prince charming. He was handsome and intelligent. Suddenly, someone was very interested in Tina romantically. Their relationship progressed rapidly and they began to talk of marrying as soon as they both graduated.

Tina had never been sexually active before. She felt trapped in her emotional turmoil of wanting to delay intercourse until marriage and wanting to experience sexual intimacy with her future husband. Soon they were alone and the decision was made. Tina gave herself completely. The first time that they had intercourse, she became pregnant.

Tina's Dilemma

Tina had always said that she was pro-life. In fact, she had done a research paper on the subject during her freshman year. Now, however, she was confronted with a pregnancy that would change her life. She wanted to complete her education, and she and her fiance wanted to become established in their professions. They agreed to abort the pregnancy and to wait until it was convenient to have their children.

Fertility Crisis

I saw Tina three years later as an infertility patient. Her engagement had broken; she had not married her college sweetheart. After college in her workplace, Tina met Will, another wonderful man. They were married and had been trying to conceive for over a year. Tina told me that Will did not know about her previous pregnancy and abortion. "He would not understand and might be very angry," she explained.

Tina was experiencing difficulty sleeping, nightmares, poor appetite and inability to achieve orgasm. She had obviously never confronted her emotions about having the abortion and was overwrought with guilt. My attempt to convince Tina to discuss all of this with Will fell on deaf ears.

A fertility evaluation indicated no male-factor problems. An X-ray study to determine whether Tina's fallopian tubes were blocked (hysterosalpingogram) showed that both were open and not obviously damaged by infection. Tests indicated that Tina was not ovulating regularly, possibly as a result of the extreme stress she was experiencing.

Tina's Recovery

After several sessions in the office, Tina decided that she must tell Will about her past in order for her to be able to move forward and to experience emotional and spiritual healing. I reminded her of my breakthrough as I obeyed God and decided to "live the truth," including confessing to some pretty difficult past failures. When she told Will, instead of rejection and humiliation, Tina found forgiveness, love and acceptance. Her depression is resolving. Tina's sexual response to Will is improving. Her appetite is returning, and I trust that a pregnancy will soon follow.

Reflections and Perspectives

by Donald M. Joy

I found myself listening to a case much like Tina's. Betty revealed that Bill didn't even want to talk about their high school senior year abortion. Here was her presenting problem:

"My high school sweetheart and I had the exact same experience as Tina. We thought we were 'the same as married,' since we knew we were going to get married as soon as we could. But we were unable to get married until two years after we graduated.

"Bill and I never told anyone about our abortion, and we were sure that when we had other children we would forget the pain of the senior year abortion. Why is it that with each new baby I experience a terrible grief? I often tear up when I'm nursing a baby or changing a diaper. Is something wrong with me? When I want to talk with Bill about my feelings he clams up and says he doesn't want to talk."

Betty and her husband went through a terrific stress at seventeen. As you read Tina's case you have to suspect that most "post abortion stress" couples break up. Post-traumatic stress disorder (PTSD) symptoms also follow most premature first intercourse cases, even when there is no pregnancy or abortion. The stress of ending the courtship relationship with intercourse without moving into a lifelong unconditional commitment with publicly sanctioned marriage traumatizes and breaks most premature first intercourse relationships. The pair bond that has been formed constitutes one new combined persona which is now tragically abused as it struggles to survive without the security of marriage.

PTSD is defined by the *Diagnostic and Statistical Manual of Mental Disorders,* 1987, in this way:

> The person has experienced an event that is outside the range of usual human experience that would be markedly distressing to almost anyone, e.g., serious threat to one's life or physical integrity; serious threat or harm to one's children, spouse, or other close relatives and friends; sudden destruction of one's home or community; or seeing another person who has recently been, or is being, seriously injured or killed as the result of an accident or physical violence.

Some of the standard symptoms of the PTSD are: anxiety, emotional isolation, sleep disturbance such as nightmares, impaired memory, trouble concentrating (intrusive thoughts and memories), survival guilt, depression, drug or alcohol abuse, eating disorders, anniversary reactions and spiritual numbing.

Several of these symptoms are reported in Tina's medical case, and Betty also suffered from several of them. When trauma strikes, Betty may find some comfort in seeing how blessed she and Bill are to have passed through the trauma together and to have survived reasonably well.

For those couples who break up, as most do after premature intercourse, after an out-of-wedlock pregnancy or after an abortion, most of the individuals move on to a series of future relationships. In virtually all cases, they are so devastated by the lost love that they tend to become quickly sexual with each partner, without the patient building of a pair bond. These multiple-partner people then often find that they have accidentally laminated sexual pleasure to "temporary" and "no responsibility" relationships. They do not bond deeply in marriage with its reality of tough life experiences day after day. They are highly vulnerable to having an affair which offers pleasure without responsibility.

It is not surprising that Bill is unwilling to discuss his feelings about the abortion. His sterling quality shows up in his sticking with Betty through the pregnancy, the abortion and in entering what must be a very good marriage. But the male brain is organized in such a way that most men are not easily able to put their feelings into words. I report on this fetal brain development difference in my *Bonding* book, Chapter Five. Bill could tell his story to a trusted confidant, but the secret now of a decade or more is still eating away at his integrity.

So, Betty and Bill are the rare and lucky couple. They have each other and a family of healthy children. But, as with the case of Jamie and David in Chapter Seven, it is important to give themselves permission to grieve. I suggest that they find a pastor or a Christian counselor who can help them, even now, to revisit the scene of the abortion decision, to name that baby which has become so real in guilt-sealed memory, and to accept the forgiveness that comes from a full disclosure before God and one or two very trusted and forgiving people.

The bottom line is that after an abortion the grief continues for a very long time. Healthy grieving faces the truth and shares it in confession and true repentance, Then it moves through stages of anger, the regret of bargaining and trying to justify or to get another chance, then substantial depression before the breakthrough to acceptance. When grief has ripened, they will be able to comfort and support people who have been traumatized by premature sex, pregnancy, abortion and any number of painful losses. So it is important for Betty and Bill to get on with their good grief. I explore their case more extensively in my book, *Re-Bonding*.

I find it hard to believe that Dr. Hager encouraged, maybe even insisted, that Tina tell her husband about her abortion. I thought there were some secrets that everybody needs to keep.

There are a couple of reasons why sexual secrets need to be aired with one's spouse.

First, we all have a sense that sharing sexually is the ultimate vulnerability and joining of spirits with another person. When we have become naked and unashamed in pairs, we have no more visible, anatomic secrets: We know as we are known. This ultimate bonding experience seals the secrets. If either person ever gossips and tells about the sexual intimacy, the bond is virtually shattered by that exposure of secrets. So the first reason for sharing is that sexual history will reveal the brokenness of our past efforts at finding human fulfillment through sexual vulnerability and sharing. The bonding effects are ultimate and final even without penetration or pregnancy. It is the "ultimate nakedness" which laminated two spirits to a sharing of secrets which constituted a new secret, one new persona, the "couple." Marriage is entered on a firm foundation when the secrets are shared.

A man named John asked me anxiously one day whether Andrea's spontaneous confession to having had an abortion during her recent engagement demanded that he tell all and reveal that he had produced an abortion when he was 16.

"There's no demand," I offered, "but she has given you a wonderful opportunity to clear the deck of the ghosts from your past sexual misadventures."

Later, I served as the officiating clergyman for their wedding. In my final premarriage session with them, I congratulated them.

"John and Andrea," I began fairly formally just before we closed with prayer, "I congratulate you for creating a solid foundation for this marriage. You each

brought in the bulldozers and leveled the remaining ruins of your past relationships. The now conquered debris that you have put under foot will be a solid base for your marriage. You have done good work!"

The second reason for telling the secrets is that sexual response is a very fragile part of an intimate marriage. Women tend to be more easily inhibited from orgasmic response by past sexual memories than men. A woman's sexual response system is sometimes called a "para-sensory" system, because it resides in a complex "envelope" of her present feelings about everything in general, about her man in particular, her hormonal and general physiologic condition and her levels of fatigue and stress. A young man, in contrast, is fired by hormones. He is specifically and precisely focused on genital pleasure, now! By mid-career, however, a man tends to become more complex in his sexual response. So at mid-life, unresolved secrets and distracting memory of long buried shame often complicate even the husband's response.

Here are some rules that could govern whether and when to tell one's secrets to a fiance or a spouse:

1. Share the secret as a way of clearing the air for complete truth in the one new persona pair bond.
2. Share the secret as a way of inviting the partner to help you deal with past shame and guilt.
3. Do not share the secret as a way to dump your problems on your spouse.
4. Do not share explicit details which would only torment your partner. Resist the partner's probing, because vivid images you create in your partner may actually create your ghost in your spouse's memory.
5. Do not share details which incriminate previous partners, unless criminal proceedings need to begin against them. Those former partners deserve to make their own peace in their journey toward integrity and deliverance from shame and guilt. "Confess your own sins," is a good rule in every case, "not those of others."

Sharing of secrets is healthiest when it is voluntary, timed by the yearning for establishing or maintaining a marriage in which no ghosts haunt the bedroom or any aspect of the relationship.

You will find other guidelines on telling the truth in any of the many Twelve Step recovery programs. Paul Pearsall in his recent best seller, *Super-Marital Sex: Loving for Life*, reports on research with a thousand couples over a 10-year period. Among his most striking findings was the need for complete honesty in pursuit of a "super marriage." He begins by asking the partners to reconstruct what they would call their "super senseless sex secret," and imagine the relief that they would have if their partner understood that silly, stupid or tragic piece of their history.

In this chapter we have looked at Tina's post-abortion journey, complicated by infertility. We have reflected on the common painful experience of millions of us who have had to work through "post traumatic stress disorder." In a marriage, the very best recovery resources we have are in that intimate sharing that becomes possible in an ultimately honest marriage.

Chapter Ten

Baseball vs. Europe

by W. David Hager, M.D.

As we grow and mature, we pride ourselves in our ability to make our own decisions. Many issues are decided for us when we are children and teenagers. Our parents make decisions about what clothing we will wear, whether to have braces for our teeth or corrective eye surgery for a lazy eye, what schools to attend and whether to attend church.

When I was about 15-years-old, my family planned a summer trip to western Europe. My parents were elated about the opportunity for our entire family — father, mother, brother Dan and sister Nela — to experience this event together.

I was playing Babe Ruth League baseball that summer and made the All-Star team. The tournament games would be held during the time that the trip was planned. In my adolescent maturity, I decided that I would not go with the family so that I could play baseball with my friends. My parents were very low-key about the potential controversy. They quietly went ahead and made their plans including acquisition of my passport and tickets.

Two weeks before the trip, a family meeting was called, and I was informed that the long-term value of the trip exceeded the benefits I could gain from playing baseball. They announced that I would be accompanying the rest of the family to Europe.

My initial reaction was one of disbelief. I wanted to make my own decision about my plans. My parents realized that at 15 I had not lived long enough to know in every case which decision would be in my best long-term interest. Reluctantly, I went on the trip, and as you can imagine had one of the most rewarding experiences of my life.

Not all decisions made for us are rewarding. Sometimes choices have to be made for us to protect us from ensuing danger or even from ourselves. Worse yet, sometimes we are so distracted that somebody else simply has to make the best decision they can for us. The story of Toni and the loss of her ovaries is one of these tragic episodes in which Tony was unable to make a decision that would affect the rest of her life.

Case #10

The Loss of Ovaries:
Toni's Tragedy

Toni was a 16-year-old, single young woman when she was brought to the emergency room with complaints of fever, chills and severe abdominal pain. She had not been feeling well for five days, but she did not seek medical care. She was nauseated and had been unable to keep food down for three days. She was doubled up in pain and was extremely difficult to examine because her pain was so severe. Toni had a temperature of 103 degrees, her pulse was 120 and an ultrasound scan revealed a large mass in the pelvis with free fluid in the abdominal cavity consistent with a ruptured pelvic abscess — an infected mass involving the uterus, tubes and ovaries.

Toni's History

Toni had initiated sexual activity at 15 years of age with her 17-year-old boyfriend. She felt that they had a wonderful relationship, and they had discussed marriage in the future. Toni was certain that they were mutually monogamous. Toni's father and mother worked hard to make ends meet and to provide a good home for their three children, but because they both worked so hard at their vocations, there was little time devoted to open communication and sharing of experiences.

Toni and her siblings were in daycare in their early years, and after starting school they frequently were home alone without a parent in the house until after six or seven o'clock in the evening. Toni sought attention and affection and found both in a sexually active relationship.

Septic Emergency

In the hospital, Toni was judged to have a ruptured pelvic abscess. She was developing signs of septic shock where bacteria spread into the blood stream and cause the blood pressure to fall when toxic substances are released by the bacteria. I convened a long discussion with Toni and her parents. I informed them of the need for emergency surgery and of the possible need for removal of the uterus, tubes and ovaries.

Indeed, at the time of the surgery, it was determined that the abscess involving both tubes and both ovaries had ruptured and pus had spilled into the abdominal cavity. As we have mentioned, these abscesses are often initiated by gonococcal or chlamydial infection. Afterward, other bacteria, such as those that grow in the absence of oxygen, infect and cause an abscess, which is actually a walled-off mass of pus.

What Has to Go?

Reluctantly, the decision was made to remove both of Toni's tubes and ovaries. The uterus was left in place in spite of the risk of infection, in case she might want to pursue in vitro fertilization after marriage. High potency antibiotics were used to treat her infection and she recovered and did well physically. As one would expect, she was very depressed and required extensive counseling and support. Her hormones were replaced by administering estrogen orally.

Life Without Ovaries and Tubes

Toni felt that her parents had made a bad decision in allowing the surgery to be done. But she did not comprehend how ill she had been. Removal of a woman's sexual organs surgically is necessary for specific indications only. Unfortunately, those indications are not always present and yet the surgery is performed anyway.

Removal of the uterus — the womb — is called a hysterectomy. This can be completed via the abdomen or the vagina. Removal of the tubes is called a salpingectomy. Removal of the ovaries is called an oophorectomy. Both are normally done abdominally, although with the laparoscope we can now remove the ovaries transabdominally without opening the abdominal wall with a large incision.

Patients who have cancer of the uterus or ovaries, uncontrollable bleeding from the uterus, marked enlargement of the uterus from leiomyomata — fibroids — which are smooth muscle tumors or patients with severe endometriosis, which can cause severe pain and discomfort, may require removal of the uterus and possibly of the tubes and ovaries.

It is important to note, however, that with today's modern technology we can frequently treat the problem without removing the reproductive organs. Laparoscopy — using a lighted scope to look into the abdomen — enables us to visualize the problem without making a large abdominal incision. Through the laparoscope, we can direct laser beams or electrical cautery to treat endometriosis, cut adhesions and remove fibroids and ovarian cysts. New, powerful antibiotics enable us to more successfully treat severe infections and hopefully avoid scenarios like Toni's. We can also do laparoscopically-assisted vaginal hysterectomy and remove uteri vaginally, with more rapid recovery, in many cases that once could only be removed abdominally.

With new techniques of assisted conception such as in vitro fertilization, patients can conceive even with their tubes and/or ovaries removed. For this reason we leave the uterus in place if at all possible. The removal of any pelvic organ should never be taken lightly and should only be done when absolutely necessary.

Prognosis: Is there Love after Loss?

The removal of a woman's reproductive organs is not a matter to be taken lightly. Removal of the uterus extirpates an organ that is the site of the development of new life and from which monthly menstrual periods come. Removal of the ovaries takes away the site of the production of the two principal female hormones, estrogen and progesterone. In all cases there are both physiological and psychological factors to consider.

On the one hand, ovarian cancer is a very difficult disease to diagnose in its early stages, and removal of the ovaries may serve to protect those one out of seventy women who will develop this form of cancer. On the other hand, removal of any of the reproductive organs may leave some women feeling that they are not the same persons they were before and shake their self esteem to its very foundation. These factors must be considered and discussed before hysterectomy and/or oophorectomy are carried out.

It is possible to replace the hormones that would be produced by the ovaries if they are removed. Both estrogen and progesterone can be administered in doses to satisfy physiologic needs, however not all women can tolerate hormonal replacement due to various side effects. Some women may still have symptoms of depression and loss of self esteem in spite of this therapy. In Toni's case oophorectomy was necessary, but we discussed all of the possible emotional and physical side effects before surgery.

Reflections and Perspectives

by Donald M. Joy

Among the painful experiences I have listened to, loss of reproductive capacity surely ranks near the top in its persistent, long-term grief and sense of loss. Here is one situation I've heard:

"Toni's story is much like mine, only my mother sent me for an abortion at 16 and secretly arranged for the doctor to do a complete hysterectomy on me disguising the whole thing as the abortion. At 40, how can I sort out my anger at my mother, my rage at being deprived of my gift of fertility and affection and wondering what these synthetic hormones I'm taking are really doing to me?"

Following is a brief description of the counsel I offered this individual.

The first two issues — anger at your mother and your anger at the removal of your reproductive system — are closely related. The third is a medical question complicated by your own emotional state.

Let me just state what is obvious to all of us, I think. When we manufacture a chemical that replaces some natural chemical produced in our bodies, it will not work in exactly the same healthful way that our body's natural chemicals work. So I would recommend that you work with a physician who will help you calibrate the dosage and the actual synthetic hormone which gets the best results for you. These, I am told, often vary from one manufacturing source to another.

Your anger at your mother will be a fully orbed rage until you do careful grief work on your lost reproductive system. Let me walk you through a strategy for grieving. Then I'll come back to the issue of anger at your mother.

1. Take time to count the losses.

I find that with major losses it is urgent to write them down, study them, decide what is gone forever and list every detail as if it were your inventory written from the sidewalk as you surveyed the burned ruin of your home. When you contemplate how much of your identity is wrapped up in your sexuality and fertility, you will be giving yourself permission to do long-term grieving.

2. Decide what you have left that has value.

If you had lost a leg, you could begin to see that there are ways to compensate for the loss. In the same way, it is important for you to ask how you can compensate for the loss of your fertility and your sense of being a woman. Write a list of your favorite ways to invest time — the ways that make you feel valuable, competent and respected. Many women and men lose the high voltage sexual energy of their youth when they reach the fifth or sixth decades of life, but find that their identity is not profoundly dependent on their sexual prowess or their reproductive capacity. If you can identify some identity issues which bring you a great sense of pleasure and status, you will see a shaft of light shining in your darkness.

3. Deal with the Mother issue.

You may choose to forgive her. If so, be sure that you take a few years to count your losses and strike a posture to make life worthwhile without the reproductive organs she ordered removed. In the meantime, it will be important to get some emotional space between yourself and your mother. As an adult, it will be helpful to put physical distance between you as well while you are doing the grief inventory. This is likely to last during the normal motherhood years and beyond. It is healthy to report to her that you need the distance since her choice has set your life-long agenda, and you need to sort out what it means to you.

Grief begins with denial. Your period of denial passed quickly. As a teen-ager, you soon were aware that something had gone wrong.

The second layer of grieving is anger. Elizabeth Kubler-Ross found the five stages of grief as she worked with dying people. These five stages also show up in the ways we handle other major losses. The best place to put anger is on paper. I urge people to get it all out and to seal it up to keep while the rage cools down.

The third layer of grief is bargaining. Many of us want a miracle, restored reproductive organs! But that is an appeal to magic and is actually a fantasy. You can yo-yo right back into denial when you lose touch with the reality of your permanent loss. But bargaining replays the past, tracing the possible points at which earlier choices led to the present crisis. So bargaining is a useful time of review. It can get morbid, however, and place significance on irrelevant cause- effect relationships.

Bargaining moves us into depression. Healthy depression means we have faced the truth: the long-term effects of the loss. In the depression phase of healthy grieving, we have a distinct sense of clean sadness. It is clean because we have done our sorting out work first, and we have faced the fact that life on this planet has ended as we have known it. Only then can we move on to the final stage of grieving: acceptance.

You will know that your grief work has paid off when you find a zest for your revised vision of life, of yourself and of your future. Only then can you really contemplate the needs of other people. Grief is an all-consuming career. But now you may even consider how your mother has handled her own guilt and shame associated with the hysterectomy into which she trapped you.

Should you choose to forgive your mother at this point, you can do it without denial and can go far beyond words. Indeed, you know you have achieved acceptance healing when you can hear yourself referring to the tragic loss as an event outside of yourself and your present emotions. You could listen as she responds to tell you what that decision did to her. And in the process you would discover for yourself what the term "wounded healer" can mean.

In this chapter, Toni's tragic emergency and the loss of her tubes and ovaries set the stage for us to examine how deeply our fertility and reproductive sexual capacity is wrapped around our identity. There is life after removal of part or all of a woman's reproductive system, but it is routed over a revised life map.

Toni and her future husband may find a technological way to get their bionic baby. My parishioner will not, though she and her husband can perhaps gather a foster and adoptive quiver full of children as one means to cut their losses.

If wisdom comes to those who suffer, then Toni and others like her are surely enrolled in a school where gold embossed diplomas are issued regularly. With her continuing expert medical care, we salute Toni and expect her to live again in some glorious life trajectory.

Chapter Eleven

Confession in a Hotel Room

by W. David Hager, M.D.

My walk as a Christian has been a persistent journey, but I have had several detours along the way. In spite of my strongest intent, I find, like Paul, that for much of my walk I was doing exactly what I did not want to be doing, then feeling like a miserable failure. I have also found that God understands my humanity even more than I do, and he has been eager to forgive me and to help me find my way back to the path of Christian maturity.

In 1990, my life had reached a plateau. I was not growing. I was spinning my feet as if I were on a treadmill. I had become aware over several months that my spiritual fog was affecting me as husband, father and physician.

I described the change in my life that began in a Washington, D.C. hotel room in Chapter Nine. Usually when I travel there, I arrive late in the evening, grab a meal and go to bed. This time, however, my secretary had made plans that landed me early in D. C., with most of a day without a specific itinerary. It was pouring rain.

I sat alone in my room with Donald Joy's book, *Unfinished Business*, my Bible and with God, who was trying to deal with me about my lack of growth in his ways.

As I read, I sensed that God was saying to me, "David, I can go no further with you until you become totally obedient to me." I knew exactly what he meant. God was calling me to total repentance, to total confession and to total obedience.

I cried out, "God, I can't do it. I can't do what you are asking. It will cost me too much. It will cost me everything that I hold dear."

In response to my argument, God said, "OK, but I cannot go any further in growth with you until you choose to be obedient to me."

I struggled with my reason and my emotions. I begged God for another way. I bargained with him, all to no avail. He demanded obedience, not some bargaining sacrifice or deal.

After several miserable hours, I got on my knees in that hotel room in deep sorrow, confessed my sins and pledged my obedience to Jesus. I felt the most amazing sensation of being clean and whole. It was a supernatural high.

In that new state of elation, I began to write. I wrote all of my feelings about the past. They simply poured out of me on to paper. As I wrote, I found God's Spirit helping me to be obedient as I honestly tried to lay everything out before him. I still had great fear of losing those dear to me, but I knew that I had to obey God in every detail.

I had suffered the consequences of my behavior for

several years, even though I was unaware that I was paying for my disobedience. Often, I conclude, people are not aware of how their choices and actions are affecting them in every way. God demands total obedience. In being obedient — in taking the blind leap off the cliff of our despair — we find God with arms open wide to catch us and to restore us. It is, after all, "in dying that we live." It is in giving up that we gain — in risking everything ,we are restored.

My patients help me at least as much as I help them. Why didn't I learn from experience that my carelessness in walking in daily obedience with God led me into the fog and arrested my growth as a mature husband, father and churchman? Wanda's case is so parallel to my blind staggering in faith that her repeated infections stand like a parable of my sin.

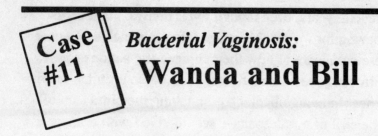

Bacterial Vaginosis:
Wanda and Bill

Wanda is a 33-year-old mother of two. She married her first husband when she was 21. They had two children within four years.

I saw Wanda in the office for a gynecologic visit. She came with complaints of vaginal discharge, vaginal itching and a distressing vaginal odor which was very embarrassing to her. I made a diagnosis of bacterial vaginosis (BV) and prescribed an oral antibiotic.

Three months later she returned with a similar infection, and I repeated the treatment. I also suggested that her husband be treated since she had such a rapid recurrence. Wanda indicated that the situation at home was not good, and that her husband was living in an apartment alone. He refused antibiotic treatment.

Repeat Diagnosis

The next time I saw Wanda, she was divorced and was dating Bill. Bill was a divorcee whom Wanda met at a party given by a mutual friend. Wanda had symptoms of vaginitis, and I found on microscopic examination of the vaginal secretions that she was suffering again from bacterial vaginosis. She was treated with metronidazole, an antibiotic that is usually effective in curing this infection.

Over the course of the next two years, Wanda continued to be sexually active with Bill and continued to have episodes of BV. Treatment would alleviate her symptoms temporarily until she had intercourse again. Bill finally agreed to see a urologist and was found to have an infection of his prostate gland. He was treated with tetracycline and his prostatitis resolved. Wanda was treated a final time and has since had no further infections.

Treatment of BV

Bacterial vaginosis is one of the three principal types of vaginitis. The others are candida or yeast infections and trichomoniasis. The number of cases of BV is unknown, but it is thought to be more frequent than trichomoniasis which occurs three and a half million times per year in the United States. This vaginal infection is caused by bacteria which grow best in the absence of oxygen. Over the years, there has been a great debate over what bacterium causes BV. Current data indicate that bacteria called *Gardnerella vaginalis* and *Mobilluncus* species are the principal causes.

These bacteria may or may not be sexually transmitted. It is possible for a woman to be infected and her sexual partner not to be infected, although BV usually occurs only in sexually active women.

It is not uncommon for men and women to have their own particular set of bacteria on and in the genital organs. This is called the person's normal flora. When two persons have intercourse, those bacteria may be exchanged and each can potentially infect the other. This phenomenon is frequently seen when a person chooses a new sexual partner, such as renewing sexual activity after a divorce or separation. Wanda acquired her first bacterial infection from an unfaithful husband. Her infections with Bill resulted from exposure to a new flora of bacteria in a man who had a prostate infection.

Treatment and Prognosis

Fortunately, BV can be treated with antibiotics. The same antibiotic that is used to treat trichomoniasis, metronidazole, is the treatment of choice for BV. The dosage is 500 mg. twice daily for five days. Clindamycin 300 mg. orally, three times daily has also been used as an effective treatment. There are also new vaginal preparations of these antibiotics. When a woman is treated and responds, but then recurs with resumption of intercourse, her sexual partner should be treated. Men are often treated with tetracycline rather than metronidazole.

Bacterial vaginosis causes vaginal discharge, a fishy odor and discomfort. Fortunately, BV does not cause severe long term consequences. There is an association between this infection and infection after delivery among pregnant women who had these organisms in the vagina at the time of delivery. Women infected with BV at the time of surgery are at increased risk of post-opeerative infection. The use of latex condoms may be beneficial in avoiding contact with the infecting bacteria.

Not all STDs have tragic and destructive outcomes. Some, such as BV, can be effectively treated without leading to the development of serious damage to the reproductive system. All STDs, however, result in some form of discomfort or adverse symptoms. We continue

to face the spiritual truth that we can be assured of forgiveness if we seek God in humble repentance, but we
have no guarantee that we will not have to deal with the
consequences of our choices and our behavior.

Reflections and Perspectives

by Donald M. Joy

Dr. Hager seems to speak so matter of factly about a divorced woman being sexually active. I have been there, and I know how devastating it has been for me to go to bed with a date. There is a lot of pressure for previously married women to be sexual almost at once. What can we do?

The STD fear is not enough to keep most people from premature, non-marital sex. The STD scare, especially with AIDS as a threat, is provoking some celebrated playboys to demand HIV screening before dating. With all of the non-marital sex that is going on, the laboratories would be kept busy with pre- sexual STD testing if everybody tried to get responsible or be safe.

But your question probes a more profound issue well beyond "safe sex." The emotional anguish of sex without permanent and public marriage comes at a high price for both women and men. I work with singles groups across the country, so let me summarize some of the things they tell me are useful strategies:

1. Avoid the "date scene" until you are ready to pursue and close in on marriage with a well-known partner.

2. Join a singles' ministry group that is committed to a covenant of celibacy and sanctity. This means that they are openly committed to "no sex outside of marriage" and the motivation is personal in-

tegrity or holiness (living life according to the Creator's design).

3. Move socially only in non-date groups. Everybody needs social contact, but no one will be helped by sexual contact without a public marriage covenant. Preferably in odd numbered groups of non-matched partners, arrange social events: concerts, recreation, or holidays in publicly visible non-paired groups of healthy people. Only in this environment can the first six steps of pair bonding occur healthily. After Step Six (intimate kissing) the pair needs some privacy for conversation, but will be damaged by genital contact before Step Ten, the first in the set of three which I call "naked and unashamed." You can explore the bonding sequence in *Bonding*, or in my book for young women, *Celebrating the New Woman*, or my book for young men, *Becoming a Man*.

4. Refuse to date as a pair until social development has occurred in group-witnessed environments.

5. While dating, go for public places and avoid absolute privacy. If either person has had previous sexual experience, absolute privacy predicts premature absolute intimacy: sexual intercourse.

The emotional erosion of repeated sexual pairing without marriage may desensitize and harden you so that you will be unable to care deeply and constructively for anyone. Or you may develop a sexual appetite which finds maximum pleasure only in no responsibility partnerships. When the second pattern appears, marriage tends to turn dull, and an affair becomes very attractive. Promiscuity is a form of addiction and the result of compulsive behavior of any kind is devastated self respect. The machisma woman and the macho man both put on a beautiful and handsome front, but it is a facade hiding an interior hollowness and sense of devastation. You will want to keep integrity growing, life long. Honesty in sexual intimacy is an important and continuing issue for each of us.

Is there a cure for repeat blunderers? How can I stop my habitual, stubborn tendency to get myself into trouble?

Dr. Hager alluded in his own story at the opening of the chapter to the passage in St. Paul in which he complains that he himself was his own worst enemy.

When I want to do good, evil is right there with me. For in my inner being I delight in God's law; but I see another law at work in the members of my body, waging war against the law of my mind and making me a prisoner of the law of sin at work within my members. What a wretched man I am! Who will rescue me from this body of death? (Romans 7:21-24)

All of the family systems authorities these days seem to agree that we are all born broken, or at least are victims of childhood trauma and bear some scars of abnormality. One highly visible therapist insists that at least 96 per cent of families are dysfunctional and leave symptoms of some degree of disorder on their children.

Theologians and Bible teachers have always suggested that the effects of racial trauma have left us all "fallen" or "depraved" and "deprived." So at least the social scientists and the theologians are now in agreement.

Because of our backgrounds, we are all prone to addiction. An addiction is the way we compensate for being emotionally broken. For example, we all are vulnerable to feelings of shame and worthlessness. So we must choose between being dysfunctionally depressed or indulging in some form of self protection. We want to be seen in the best light, even if we have to invent or fake the good appearance.

As you read Dr. Hager's opening story at the beginning of this chapter, you watched him come to a terrible moment of truthfulness: accepting his own fog-bound distress as the result of his past choices. You then saw him take the liberating step when he took responsibility for his own addiction to self protection and self-will — having his own way. Finally, you read about his "supernatural high" and the sense of wholeness and freedom which followed. This empowered him to take truth-based and risky reconciling steps as he retraced his mistakes and made restitution based on confessed past failure.

The Hager story is exactly according to the Book! It has always been this way. The formula we find in 1 John reads:

> If we confess our sins, he is faithful and just and will forgive us our sins and purify us from all unrighteousness (1 John 1:9).

Then again,

> But if we walk in the light, as he is in the light,

we have fellowship with one another, and the blood of Jesus, his Son, purifies us from every sin (1 John 1:7).

Karl Menninger put all of this into his psychiatric book, *Whatever Became of Sin?* M. Scott Peck dished it out straight in *People of the Lie*, a book in which he describes a client whose incorrigible life-style did not yield until an extended session with a handful of confidants who supported the client during her confrontation of e-v-i-l as a way of life.

The Twelve Step programs are all self-help approaches to confronting addictive behavior, and all of them use confession and restitution and the supporting care of trusted peers as the basis of healing. So, take your choice, but the way out of our contradictory, self-destructive way of being is a painful and long-term path. But it is worth beginning now.

In this chapter, Dr. Hager has opened his own closet of personal spiritual transformation and compared it to a case of persistent bacterial vaginosis. This chronic and embarrassing disease has become our parable for dealing with a wide range of self-indulging and self-willed life style pathologies. But the cure of BV and the cure for sin continue the metaphoric exchange, as all of us try to embrace integrity and wholeness.

Epilogue

A Salute to Heroic Women!

by W. David Hager, M.D., and Donald M. Joy, Ph.D.

We stand in awe of women!

We salute you because you are part of that sublime mystery — created in the "image of God." We want to count some of the ways that we are intrigued by women:

1. Your substantial commitment to everything that matters most: to relationships, to families, to communities, to God.
2. Your gift of emotion, feeling and the whole range of convictional attachment to ideas, beliefs, causes and dreams.
3. Your instinct to mother, to organize, to manage and to wrap it all in yourself until whatever you touch becomes an extension of yourself.

Women as Vulnerable and Courageous Risk Takers

A woman seems to be at more severe risk of things going wrong in the human reproductive system. So, while we are saluting you, we also want to bless you and to name the greater risks you often bear.

You embark on nine months of uncertainty to create a child.

You give us children from the edge of anguish.

You carry your children in your heart from conception until death separates you from them; they are always especially yours.

Women Are Special to God

God made a bride of an unlikely people he described in Ezekiel 16: 6-8 as a foundling, abandoned baby girl:

> Then I passed by and saw you kicking about in your blood, and as you lay there in your blood I said to you, "Live!" . . . You grew up and developed and became the most beautiful of jewels. . . . Later I passed by, and when I looked at you and saw that you were old enough for love . . . . I gave you my solemn oath and entered into a covenant with you, declares the Sovereign Lord, and you became mine.

Israel turned out to be an exemplary form of womanhood.

When a Roman soldier opened Jesus' side, the exact word is used which appears in Genesis 2 as Adam's side is opened and the bride appears. So with Jesus' death and the opened side, the Bride and Body of Christ — the Church — appears. She is described again in the futuristic vision of Revelation 21:2:

> I saw the Holy City, New Jerusalem,
> coming down out of heaven from God,
> Prepared as a bride beautifully dressed for her husband.

We are churchmen, devoted servants to the Greatest Lady of all. We expect to be milling in the crowds of folks at that eternal Wedding Supper of the Lamb when Christ the Husband and Christ the Bride are united with their newborn children witnessing the celebration on the banks of the River of Life:

"For the wedding of the Lamb has come,
and his bride has made herself ready.
Fine linen, bright and clean,
was given her to wear. . . ."
"Blessed are those who are invited to the
wedding supper of the Lamb" (Revelation 19:7-9).

If You Found Yourself in This Book. . . .

In this book we have described the physical, emotional and spiritual consequences of the most frequently occurring sexually transmitted diseases. You may find yourself in one of several categories as you read. You may never have been sexually active outside of marriage and intend to continue a life of fidelity. You may have been sexually active prior to marriage, or have had an affair while married and are now committed, refusing to become involved outside of your marriage again. You may have had one or more sexual partners, but have no plans for marriage at this time. Wherever you find yourself, we hope you found wisdom that will be useful to you. God has made a way to deliver us from our own darkness and the darkness around us. You can read about that in Colossians 1:13-14.

For he has rescued us from the dominion of darkness
and brought us into the kingdom of the Son he loves,
in whom we have redemption, the forgiveness of sins.

God is ready to forgive us when we confess our sins to
him. You can read the guidelines in 1 John 1. We have
found that we must be obedient to God in everything
that he shows us — giving up whatever he cannot ap-
prove and accepting his way of living. Obedience is the
only path to integrity and victory over sexual failure.

If you have had a sexually transmitted disease, you
must forgive yourself and immediately take action to
avoid future infection by being monogamous within marriage or abstinent without and by insisting that your
spouse or partner do the same. An STD does not have to
ruin your life. You may need to use condoms as a con-
traceptive method or to avoid intercourse while you have
a recurrence of disease, but you can continue to thrive
sexually in a healthy marriage.

If you are suffering from the consequences of a sexually transmitted disease, remember that the harvest of
any consequence, even the worst case scenario of a ter-
minal breakdown of your immune system, does not mean
that God has rejected you or does not hear you when you
cry out for forgiveness and help. He promises restoration
of dignity and integrity, in the face of any future. And
only God can offer you two worlds of meaning, love,
and wholeness: this life and the next. And this one is
only a rehearsal! Remember?

Someone to Stand with You, Now!

Jesus is ready to stand beside you against the rejecting crowd. He once stood with an accused and shame filled woman. He faced the crowd of cynics and critics and, as you can read in the opening lines of John 8, Jesus is ready to stare them down by stooping to write unknown words in the sand of your beach. You can almost hear him saying to you, "Where are your accusers?" The crowd of your hecklers will get the message clearly from him: "We have all sinned, so let the one who is perfect cast the first insult." And you will know that they have all dropped their evil intentions and left you alone with Jesus.

Jesus is encouraging you in simple words: "Go and sin no more!" And remember, you're invited to that wedding supper as an honored guest!